The Back Pain Avenger:
Heal Chronic Back Pain and Destroy It Forever

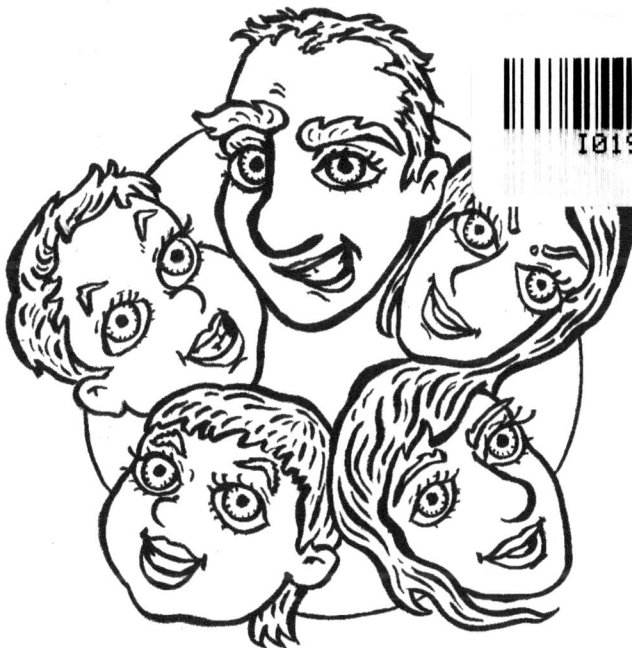

Written, illustrated, and published 2012 by Joe Chiappetta
2209 Northgate Avenue, North Riverside, Illinois, USA

Edited by Denise Chiappetta

ISBN: 978-09644323-7-6
Library of Congress Control Number: 2012902032

The book information above is the Front Matter.
The rest of this book is considered Back Matter.

http://joechiappetta.blogspot.com

Table of Contents and Discontents

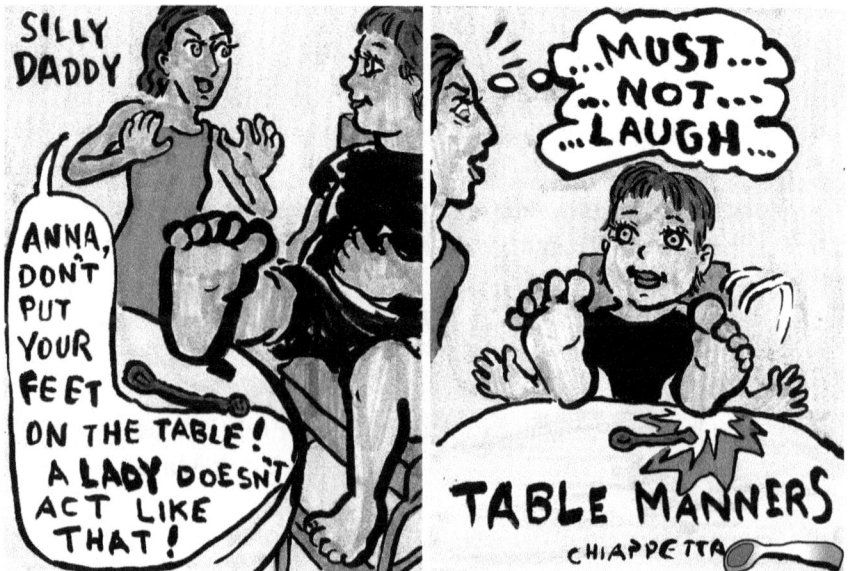

This table of contents also includes a *table of manners*.

Thank You

I would like to thank the following people whose influence has helped me to make this book more than I could have imagined:

Proofreaders: Denise Chiappetta, Lisa Fellis, David Kreydich

Role Models: Roger Parlour, Jay Shelbrack, Chris Broom, Mom, Dad

Advisers: Denise Chiappetta, Maria Chiappetta, Luke Chiappetta, Anna Chiappetta, Bill Baker, Anthony Paparo

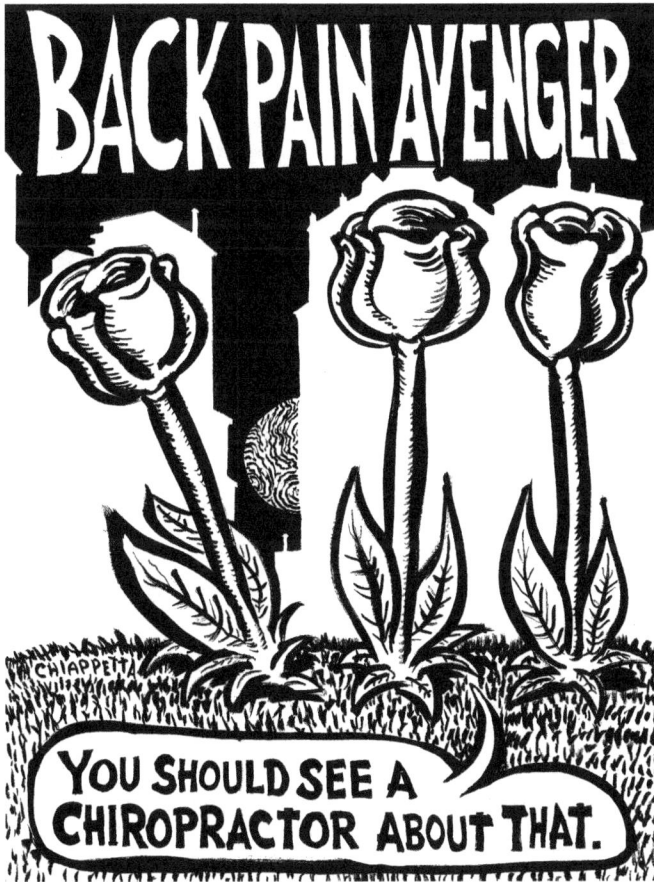

This book is partially supported by a grant from the Illinois Arts Council, a state agency.

Why I Wrote this Book

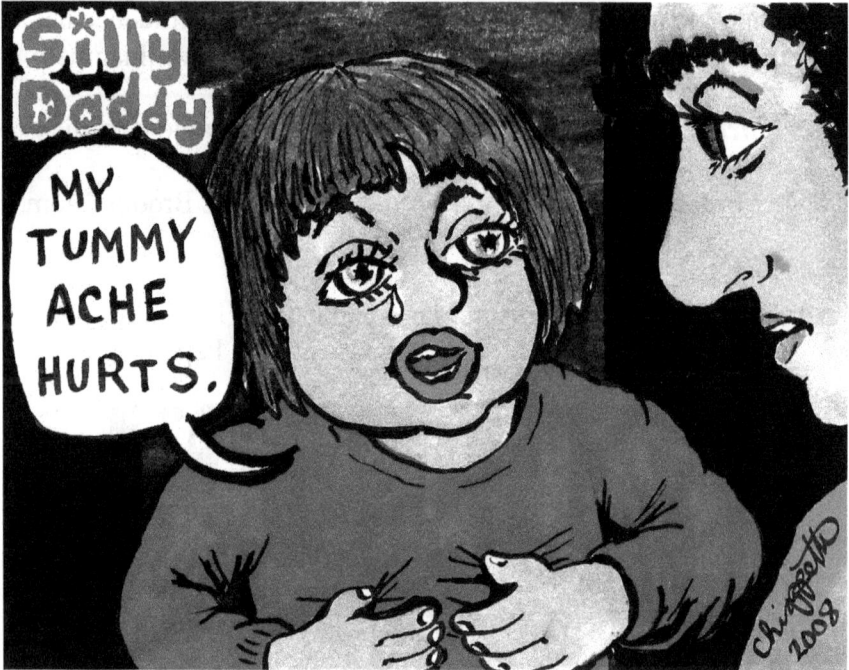

Time and time again, life turns out nothing like I expected. Five years ago, the thought of me making a book about health issues would have seemed like the dumbest, most boring thing imaginable. Moreover, I certainly never expected my growth as an artist to hit a wall. Yet that is exactly what happened when my chronic lower back pain increased to such a terrible extent that I could not sit for more than a brief period without extreme discomfort. As such, holding a coherent thought or a coherent brushstroke became a challenging experience. While I still pushed on creatively with *Silly Daddy* comics, I could feel the zeal of my cartoon communications wearing thin.

Yet it was these very trials that have led to the most amazing experience of my lifetime. Since my teenage years, I have lived with an often debilitating lower back condition, and after two decades struggling to find relief, I have finally found a rehabilitation plan that has worked completely. I wrote *The Back Pain Avenger* so that others might have the same opportunity at recovery from chronic back pain as I have had.

My intent is to share that journey with others in an educational, inspiring, and even humorous manner. Some may gloss over the disability concepts in this book and think, "It's not about me." I would amend that statement to say, "It's not about you *yet*!"

According to the US Department of Health and Human Services, 80% of Americans experience lower back pain in their lifetime. After the common cold, lower back pain is the second leading cause of lost work time, with Americans spending $50 billion each year on this condition. People are living longer and health impairments can happen to anyone at any time. Therefore, I believe

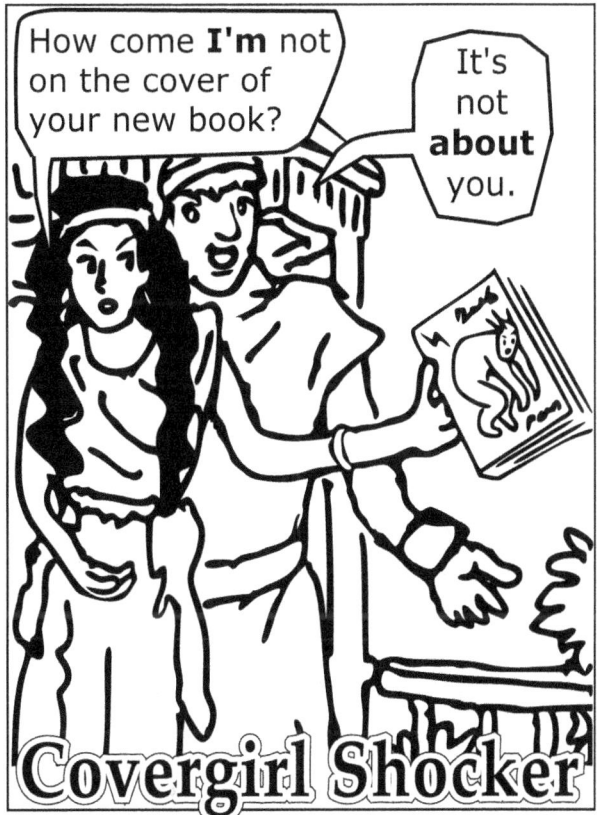

the future holds more creative exploration of disability issues for me--and perhaps for you too.

I have encountered countless people in the deepest despair of chronic back pain (self included) with no hope in sight. Since my amazing recovery in 2008, I have conversationally told these kindred spirits how I am now pain-free. To their astonishment, they eagerly want to know all the details of how I got healed. Therefore, using my twenty year background as a cartoonist and novelist, it seemed most fitting to turn those skills toward putting words and pictures together in this non-medicated memoir of my rehabilitation.

Joe Chiappetta, 2012

Chapter 1:

No Really, I'm Fine

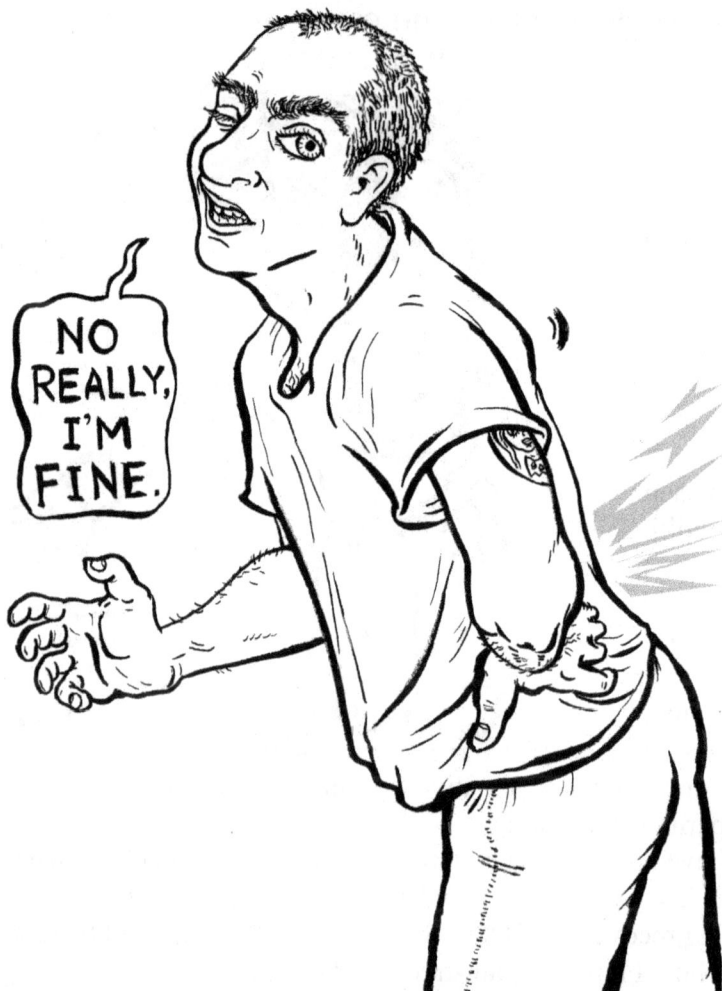

There is something about putting your life in someone else's hands that is altogether frightening and inspiring. Everyone loves to be inspired, but what about fear? I have read that perfect love drives out fear, and I believe it. My story begins in my own fearful hands and with an imperfect love. Wouldn't it be nice to jump right to the inspiring stuff? Yet that would hardly make this a true story, and my story is true. Gratefully, it ends in the hands of someone else, and with a most perfect love.

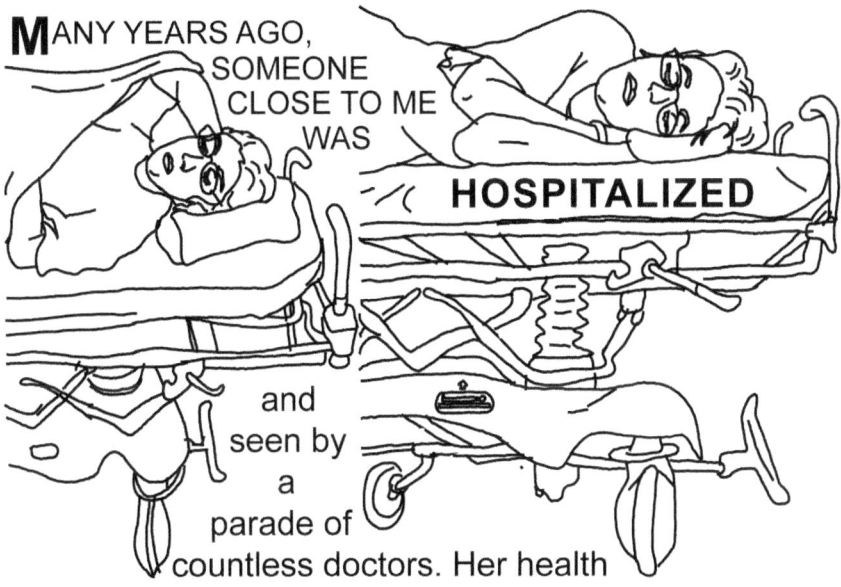

MANY YEARS AGO, SOMEONE CLOSE TO ME WAS **HOSPITALIZED** and seen by a parade of countless doctors. Her health situation was so severe, that she couldn't leave the hospital even if she wanted to. The walls were padded and the door was locked each time someone entered and exited the room. Something about being in such a room was quite intimidating. I sat by powerlessly and drew pictures. On top of all the concern I felt for her, I also had an extreme thought; "Wow, I never want to be at the mercy of hospital doctors--ever! It's like a prison. I'd rather **die**!" Helpless in the hospital? Not me.

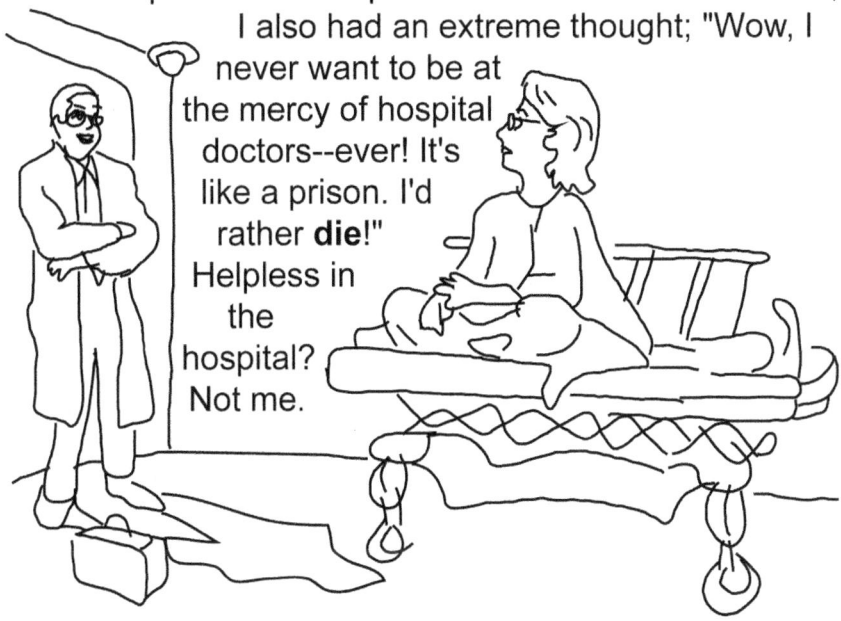

Much later, my abrupt hospital decision to "never want to be at the mercy of hospital doctors" would be put to the test. Perhaps my test could have been avoided if I had paid more attention to a simple word. It was a little term that changed the course of my life quite drastically.

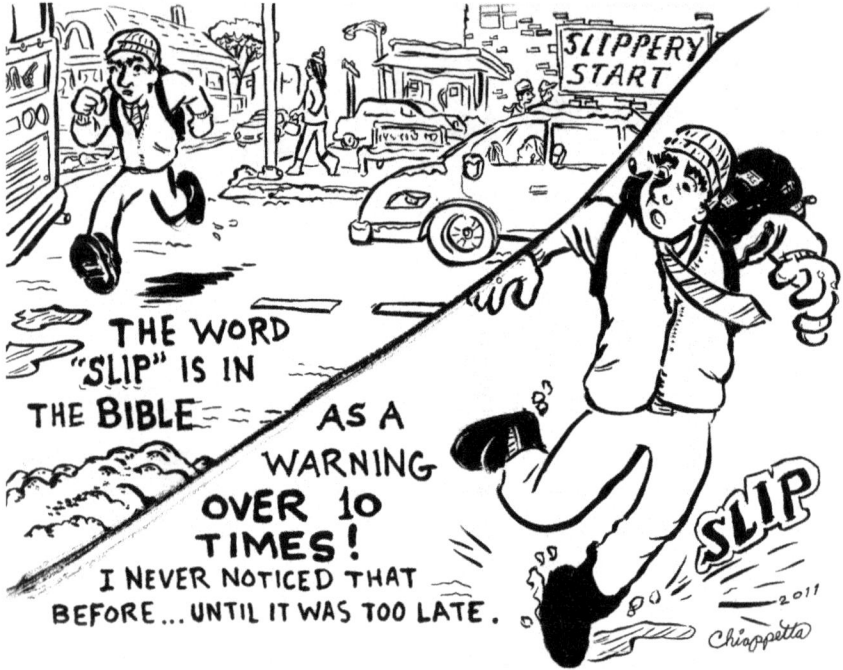

THE WORD "SLIP" IS IN THE BIBLE AS A WARNING OVER 10 TIMES! I NEVER NOTICED THAT BEFORE... UNTIL IT WAS TOO LATE.

SLIPPERY START

SLIP

Chiappetta 2011

Running across a big street named after a big former mayor of Chicago--that's where everything slipped out of control--on Cermak Road. That's when my health problems glided into a new low. I was on my way to work, trying to catch the train from Cicero to downtown Chicago. The cold winter morning hadn't affected me yet, or so I thought. I had just finished shoveling the snow by my house not twenty minutes prior.

I like Cermak Road. At the time, I was living three houses from that grand old street. For most of my life, my various dwelling places have been no more than three miles away from this major Chicago roadway. The street is named after Mayor Anton Cermak. In 1933, he took an assassin's bullet while shaking President-elect Franklin D. Roosevelt's hand, and died of those wounds a few weeks later.

As for me, no shots were fired, but I got wounded on the road that was renamed in honor of Chicago's fallen mayor. While I crossed the middle of his street, I swiftly slipped on a small unassuming patch of ice. I chalked it up to God or my many years in wrestling as to the reason why I didn't fall from this slip. I actually kept on running. Yet instantly, I knew something was seriously wrong. In roughly forty years, I had already grown somewhat accustomed to living with mild chronic back pain. However, that particular day on Cermak Road was quite different. My hip shifted ever so slightly out of control, causing a shocking and intense shooting pain to attack my lower back and not relent. In the hours, weeks, and even years thereafter, this back pain got so bad that there were times I wished I had died of my Cermak Road wounds.

Nevertheless, in automatic get-to-work mode, and with cramping, excruciating pain, I hobbled onto the train and hunched over in one of the single seats, hoping no one would ask me if I needed to go to the emergency room. It was as the train pulled out of the station toward Chicago that I had a chilling thought; "I don't think I can make it. I'm in so much pain; maybe I should just lay down right here and die. Life will go on without me. Chicago, I'm sure, will hardly miss a beat."

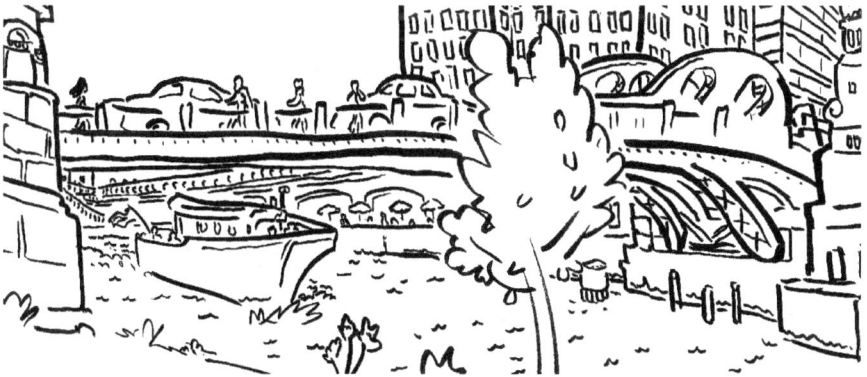

Obviously, I did not die that day. By some miracle, or sheer foolish determination, I made it to the office. However my boss, despite being legally blind, took one blurred look at my face with my hunched-over mannerism, and insisted, "Joe, you look sick. You need to go home!"

I straightened up somewhat, crafted the best smile I could fake, and made a declaration that was quite ridiculous; "No really, I'm fine."

As soon as those pitiful words jerked out of my mouth, I was overcome with a sinking familiarity; I tell people all too often that I am fine, when in reality, the exact opposite is true. This was not an

Oscar-winning performance, and my boss ran to get her boss. While she did so, I did the only thing I was capable of at the time; I lied down on the floor and closed the door to my office. Moments later, the two bosses barged into my space and insisted, "We are calling an ambulance and taking you to the hospital. Something is wrong with you! We need to get you some help."

Still wincing in pain, while clinging to the ugly gray carpeted floor, I countered, "No, I don't want to go to the hospital. I'll be fine. Just let me rest for a little while here on the floor."

"We can't do that," said the big boss. "It's a liability. Either we take you to the hospital right now, or we call you a limo right now to get you a ride home."

Not having any confidence in health professionals, which up to that point had done nothing to fix my mild chronic back pain, I attempted to sit up and act normal, like everything would blow over in a few more minutes. All the while the two supervisors said a bunch of things that I'm sure were carefully articulated to convince me to seek professional help. Yet I couldn't really focus on what they were saying. It was gibberish. My back pain was too overwhelming.

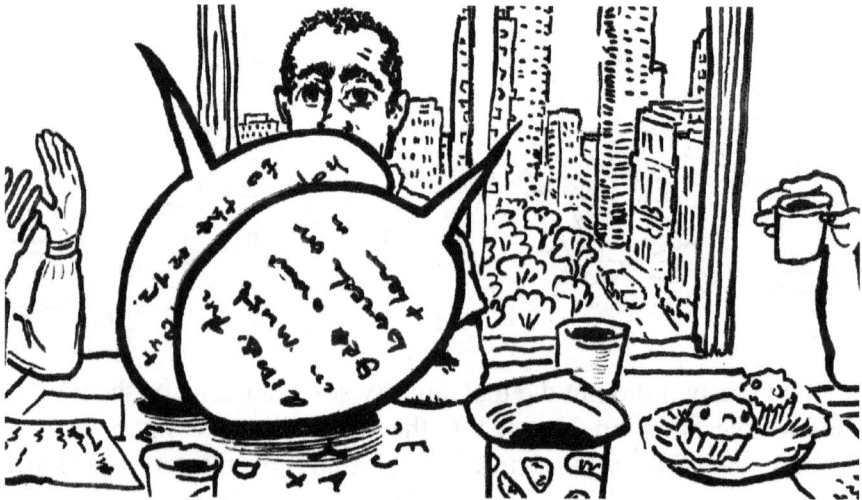

Therefore eventually I decided, "Fine, I'll just go home, but I can't afford a limo." As I started to get up, I gasped numerous times with spasms of pain.

The big boss became even more alarmed and declared, "I bet you have kidney stones. Those things are painful. Oh boy, I remember when I had mine; that was the worst experience I ever had! Don't worry about the cost of the limo. We'll pay for it."

I was too weak to tell him that I didn't think that I had kidney stones. However, I did thank him as he escorted me to the limo. While I crawled into the vehicle and lay down in the back seat, the big boss said, "Take a few days off and let us know how you're doing. But really, you need to get some help. You know us guys; we get older, and realize we're not invincible. Face the facts, Joe."

As the limo carried me home, I was determined not to end up in the hospital. I had recently been to the emergency room for an unrelated eye injury, and the thought of going back there was inconceivable.

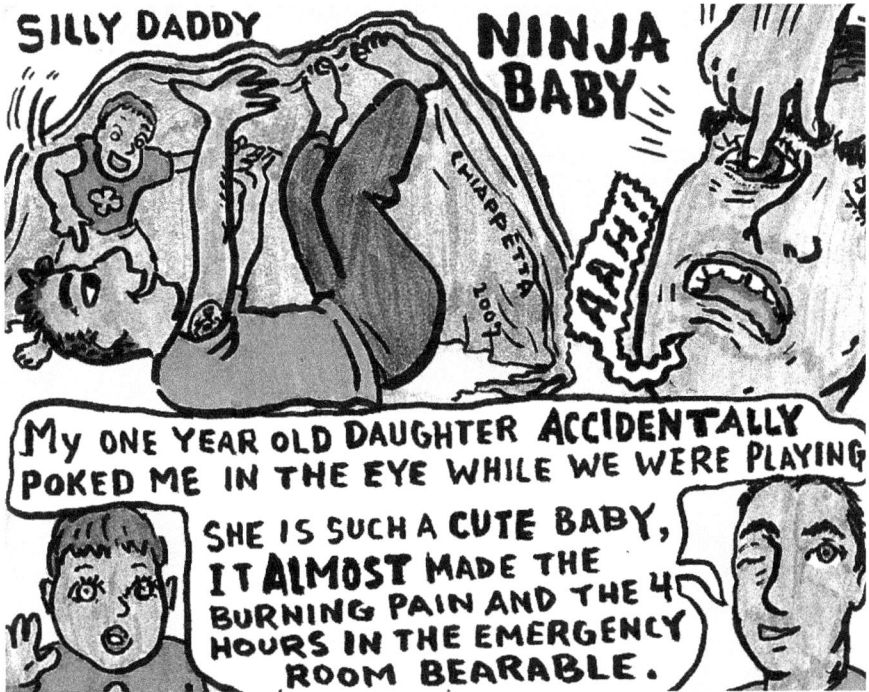

SILLY DADDY — NINJA BABY

My ONE YEAR OLD DAUGHTER ACCIDENTALLY POKED ME IN THE EYE WHILE WE WERE PLAYING

SHE IS SUCH A CUTE BABY, IT ALMOST MADE THE BURNING PAIN AND THE 4 HOURS IN THE EMERGENCY ROOM BEARABLE.

Chapter 2:

Invincible or Not

Won't someone please shed a tear for me? That would be a nice consolation, or at least I imagine it would be.

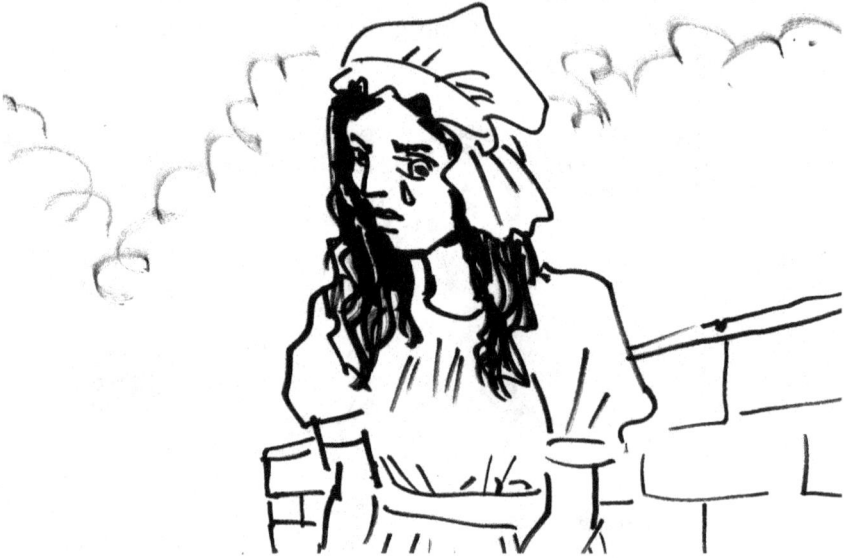

How did I get to such a state of painful existence? Let me think back. I remember younger days as a carefree parachuter, a champion wrestler, a rooftop jumper, and a fearless football player. Those were my early years--defined by the thought that my body was well-made and pretty indestructible. It all started as a child on the playground. I swung from swings with as much momentum that a seven-year-old can muster. At the highest forward arc of the swing, I would then leap off, into the warm summer sun. The moment of zero gravity as I shifted from upwards to downward was exhilarating.

Almost always, I would imagine being Spider-Man, the Beast, or any one of my favorite superheroes from the Avengers, as I came to a rolling, yet nonetheless abrupt, landing on the ground. It was just like in the Marvel Comics, or as near as I could make it out to be. The kids had a term for this daring playground activity. It was called parachuting. The problem, however, with this clever name, was that there was no actual parachute involved in the activity. Such trivial details would not serve to stop me, and I became an expert playground parachuter in no time at all.

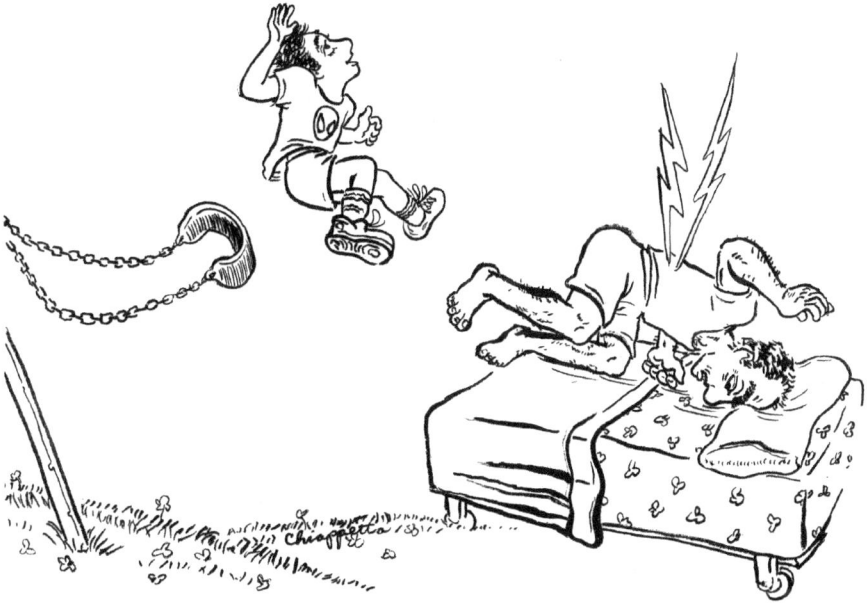

Look Mom! I'm Free-falling into CHRONIC BACK PAIN!

Thus began my pattern of causeless heroics. I would engage in related actions throughout the first two decades of my life. These activities gradually seemed to wear down my lower back. Yet the appeal of flying through the air was too strong to resist just for the sake of some adult concept called safety. If only I could have seen the bigger picture--the Cermak Road.

"Look, Mom! I'm free-falling into chronic back pain!" Quickly passing through the stratosphere, I soon landed myself more time in pain and in bed: a place known to many as the Pillow-sphere.

As far as I knew, free-fall swinging never got organized into a sport, which is where wrestling and football came in. My many seasons on the wrestling team, lifting up people from all sorts of uncomfortable positions, became part of my regular routine, as did a few seasons of gung-ho football. I was a defensive cornerback, yet couldn't catch a thing. To overcompensate for my inability to make interceptions, I recklessly attacked anyone from the other team with anything resembling a football.

This naturally landed me many big tackles, and on one occasion, a visit from some paramedics after I tackled a boy who had legs as big as a tree. I use the term "boy" loosely. While this was high-school football, I'm sure the giant running back who collided with me was made of concrete and worked in the steel mills by night. My ears were ringing from the impact with him, and I was deaf for a few minutes.

When I stumbled to my cleated feet, I kept saying, "I'm fine. Really, I'm fine." Little did I know that such a line would later become habitual. On the playing field, I must have blacked out for a brief moment, because I don't remember making that tackle. Yet when I could finally hear again, the team was patting me on the back and encouraging me for making such a fearless tackle. It apparently stopped concrete man from scoring a touchdown. The paramedics arrived to look me over. After examining my eyes and skull, they released me, saying that I didn't need to go to the hospital. Perhaps they should have been looking at my back.

Also mentionable were the occasional jumps I would take from the garage roof to the grass, just for fun. If someone were to ask me what I was thinking during those wild moments in the air, I would respond like any bird would; "I like to fly, of course." Little did I know that all that flying-high fun would give way to multiple trips to health professionals in the decades to come, and they would pluck my feathers away.

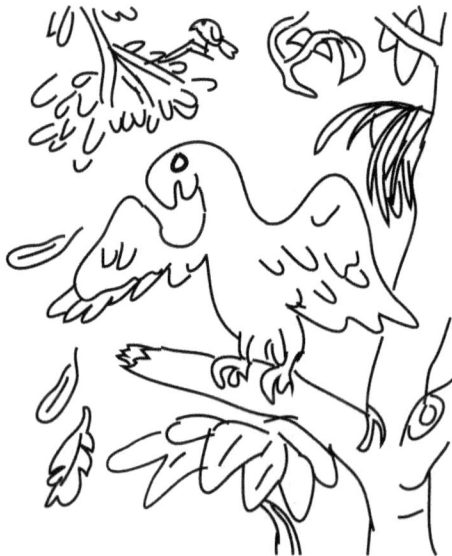

Not that I would have to wait that long. By the time I was sixteen years old, I remember my mom taking me to the doctor's office due to back pain. They x-rayed me, but couldn't find anything wrong. The best they could do was to tell me to practice proper lifting techniques. They even gave me a chart to take home so I could learn all these fancy moves. Bend at the knees, hold items close to your chest--all the usual tips. Like a good patient I adopted those proper lifting techniques to the letter. From that day onward, you would never see me lift with my back--only from the knees.

I also became very careful to always lie on my stomach whenever possible. This would relieve pressure on my lower spine and I imagined my poor overburdened discs magically recharging from the weight of the day. Lying on my stomach even became my preferred mode of playing with the kids.

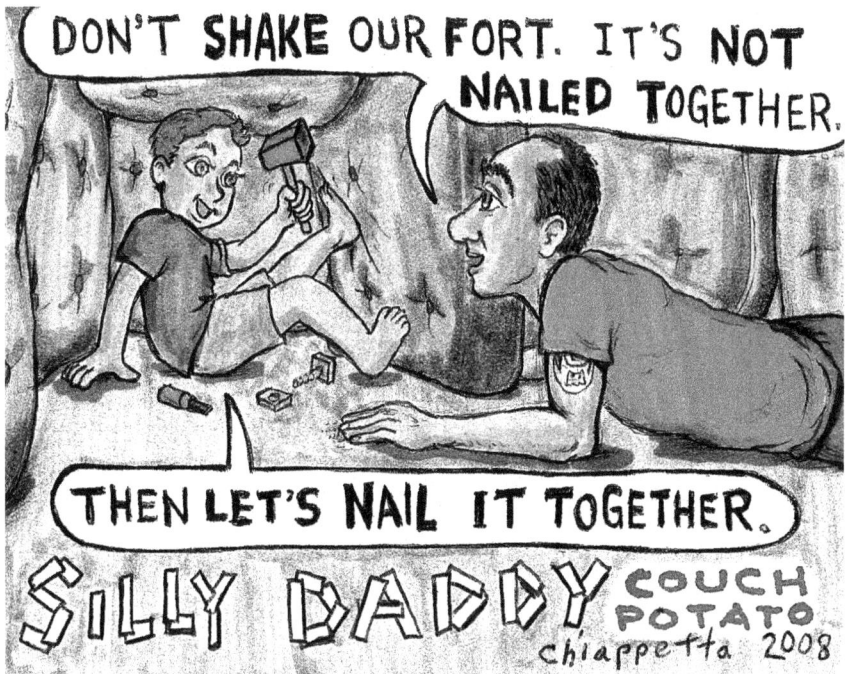

Yet proper lifting techniques and lying on my stomach never healed me. In the years that followed, other medical professionals found many things wrong with my back. The list went on and on: slightly curved spine, early stage arthritis, herniated discs, bulging discs, degenerative disc disease, not enough water in my diet, and even a neurological disorder.

A healthy back compared to my back seemed to yield medical illustrations that might make a grown man cry. It's a good thing I lack the skills to be a real medical illustrator.

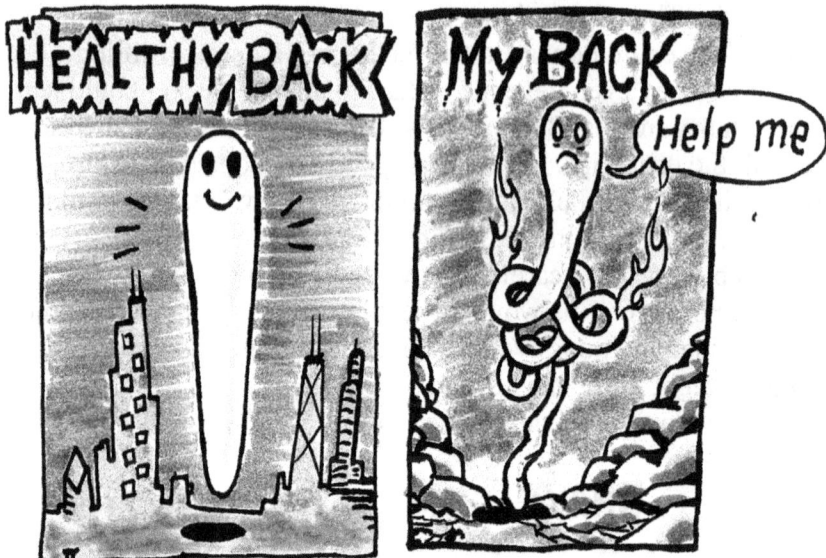

Joe Chiappetta Presents...
COPYRIGHTED MEDICAL ILLUSTRATIONS
TO MAKE YOU CRY

With the increase of these expert opinions pointing out all that was wrong with my back, I started to wonder if I was already **broken beyond repair**. If only I could find a hero to rescue me from the pains of my youth. Was there anyone who could vanquish the aching and throbbing of my lower back?

The comic books I read and collected told tales of valiance and vengeance--of the helpless everyman yanked from the clutches of injustice and death just in the nick of time. That's the kind of hero I needed. I was searching for a

Back Pain Avenger.

Chapter 3:
The Juiciest Form of Pain Relief

I have done a number of extreme and even bizarre things in an attempt to get rid of my chronic and sometimes even crippling back pain over the years. Perhaps the tangiest effort of them all was the time I used Italian Ice as a pain reliever. Yes, I am aware it's really a dessert.

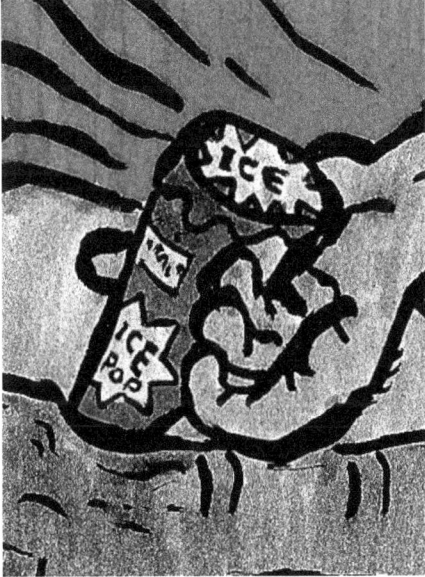

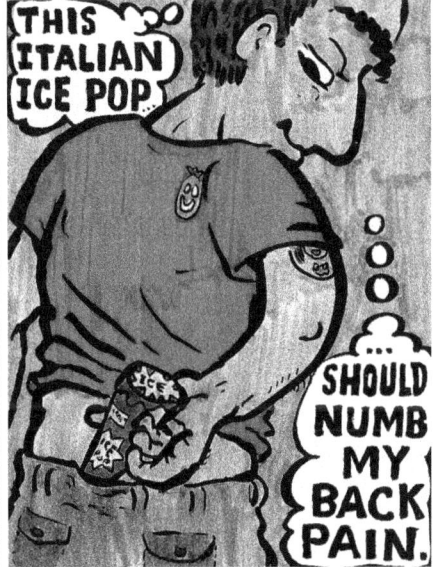

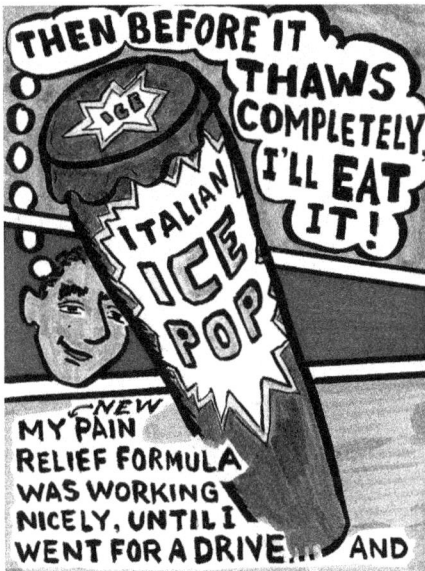

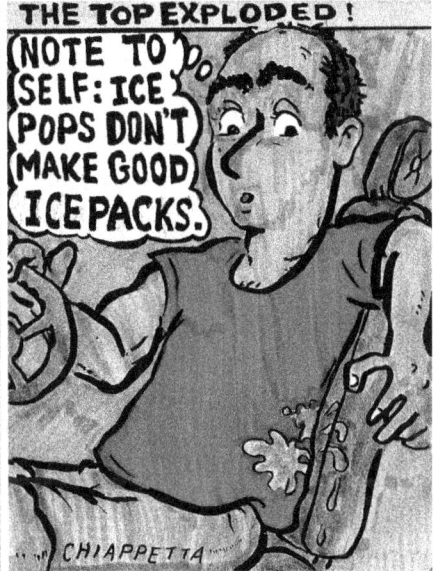

In retrospect, I'm glad to be known for serving spine-chilling laughter as the man who put a frozen snack on his lower back. My thoughts seemed logical at the time; "The innovative juices are really flowing today. While I would love to gobble this Italian Ice Pop right now, I must show a little patience. If I put the Italian Ice on my spine, it should numb my back pain. Then, before the container thaws completely, I'll eat it!"

My sweet new pain relief formula was working quite nicely. I even was feeling proud of myself for coming up with such a brilliant and utilitarian pain relief plan. Perhaps I could even market this to the physical rehabilitation community. Isn't my new procedure the kind of story that gets a person on talk shows or at least coverage in the local newspaper? The ailing everyman turns overnight sensation; surely that was my tasteful destiny!

However, my delusions of grandeur turned as sour as lemony flavor soon afterwards. I went for a car drive and the top of the Italian Ice container exploded. Italian Ice, my favorite dessert other than cookies, spilled all up and down my back in a sticky mess. "Note to self," I thought, "Ice Pops don't make good Ice Packs." This is a cold but true story of lost snackery. If it's any consolation, I made every effort to eat what little remained of that Italian Ice off of my trusty old vinyl car seat.

Humorous cruising aside, I was taking a continual beating by life due to the constant pain in my back, yet was convinced that the following proverb had little to do with me:

"Penalties are prepared for mockers, and beatings for the backs of fools." (Proverbs 19:29)

I imagined that such a proverb was there to warn other less fortunate folks who still needed to get their life in order. I presumed to be above all that. No one was actually beating my back, were they? No, I concluded. I'm a responsible, upstanding, and tax paying citizen that just happened to have developed a bad back. Yet I was determined not to let my back pain get the best of me. No solution was too out of reach. Healing I must have, no matter how foolish my quest may appear to the outside world.

Therefore, coming in at a close second place for weird pain relief escapades, was the year I spent upside down in hopes of becoming rehabilitated. Since I use the term "rehabilitation" frequently, let's first define it before I explain how and even why I would want to be upside down so much.

Definition OF Rehabilitation

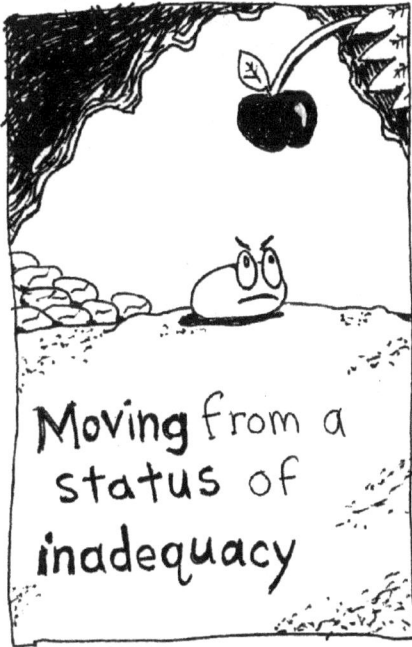

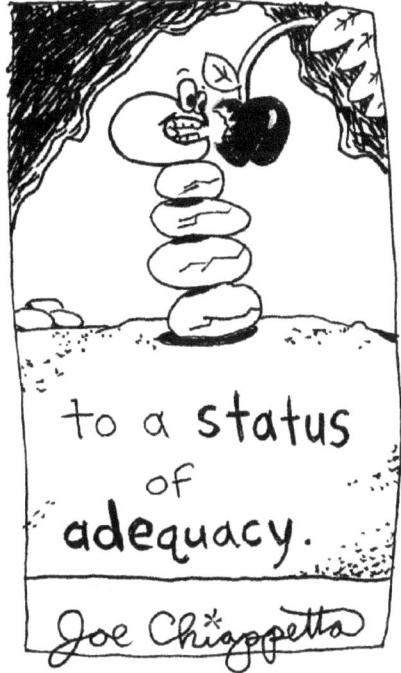

Moving from a status of inadequacy to a status of adequacy.

Joe Chiappetta

Rehabilitation is moving from a status of inadequacy in significant life areas to a status of adequacy. I realize this might not sound politically correct, but for someone who has gone through physical rehabilitation successfully, comparing my *before rehab* state of existence to my *after rehab* status, this is a most appropriate definition. For me, it was like night and day.

Done right, rehabilitation is about accomplishing goals that recover as much personal freedom, survival skills, and community involvement as possible. All in the name of rehabilitation, my chiropractor, who turned out to be no help to me at all, suggested I get an inversion table and hang upside down on it a few times a day. The theory was that this would pull apart the compressed discs in my spine and give me some much needed relief.

In no time at all, my loyal friend Roger Parlour picked up this monstrous device for me at Walmart and even assembled it. That is what friends are for--to help you turn your life around--literally. Consequently, for over a year, the inversion table took up a ridiculous amount of space in our bedroom--just ask my wife who patiently put up with all this.

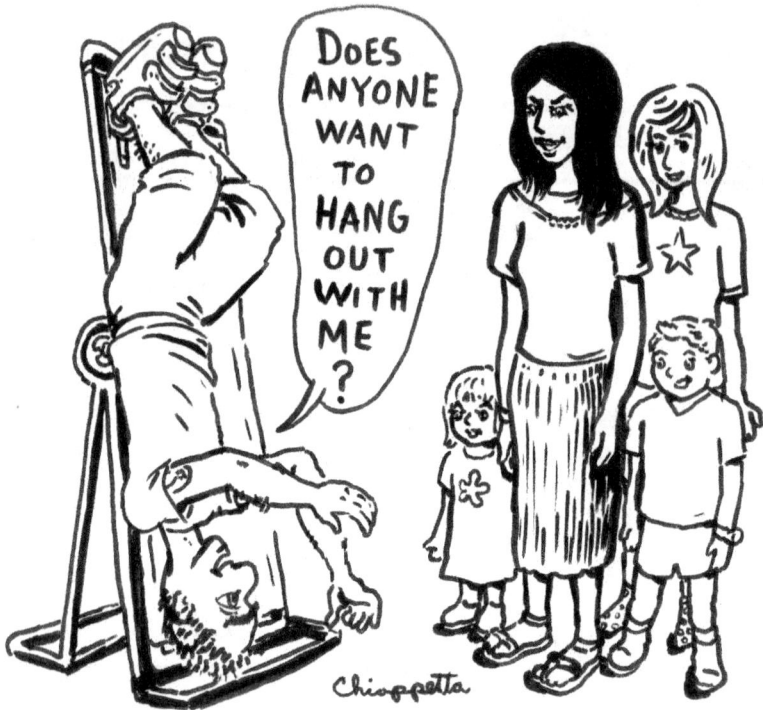

Every morning and evening I would strap my feet in position, lie back on the table, and let the device spin me over with my head just inches from the floor. I would feel instant pain relief as my entire body slowly decompressed while hanging from my feet. However, a person can't stay in this position for more than a minute. All the blood goes to your head and so you get quite nauseous. That said, I became a real pro at it, working up a tolerance so that I could hang upside down for four minutes at a time without any ill effects. Perhaps I should have been an astronaut.

From my inversion table, I would deliver all sorts of corny jokes. A favorite involved calling the family together while I was strapped in and asking, "Does anyone want to hang out with me?" Another classic cornball statement from the inversion table included an imagination of the world flipped over with gravity behaving strangely and me saying, "I'm not upside down. You are!"

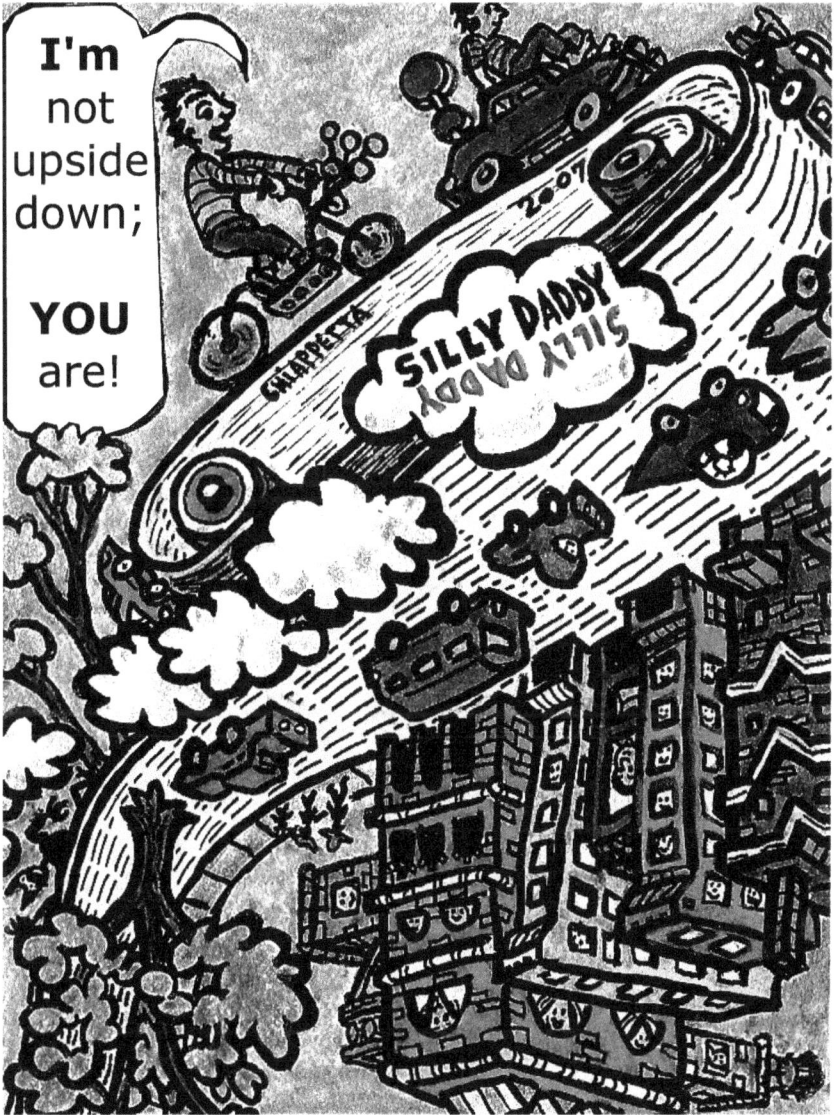

Embarrassing as it is to admit, this $250 device never actually healed me. I think my kids got the most fun out of it. I would strap in, then hold them tight and swing upside down with them, one at a time, for "safety's" sake. We would yell and scream as if falling down a great cliff on a strange adventure. I may have been disabled, but at least the kids got plenty of carnival rides out of the deal.

I discovered a few great lessons from having the inversion table. My wife loves an uncluttered bedroom. I learned that from how grateful she was when we finally got rid of the device by selling it on the Internet. I also learned that Roger, the man who set me up with the device, was a true friend. He wasn't the one who advised me to get such a contraption, but he knew, because of my back, that I physically could not go to the store, lift the device, and carry it home. That's what Roger did. He's a loyal friend, and loyalty from him and people like him continue to turn my world right side up.

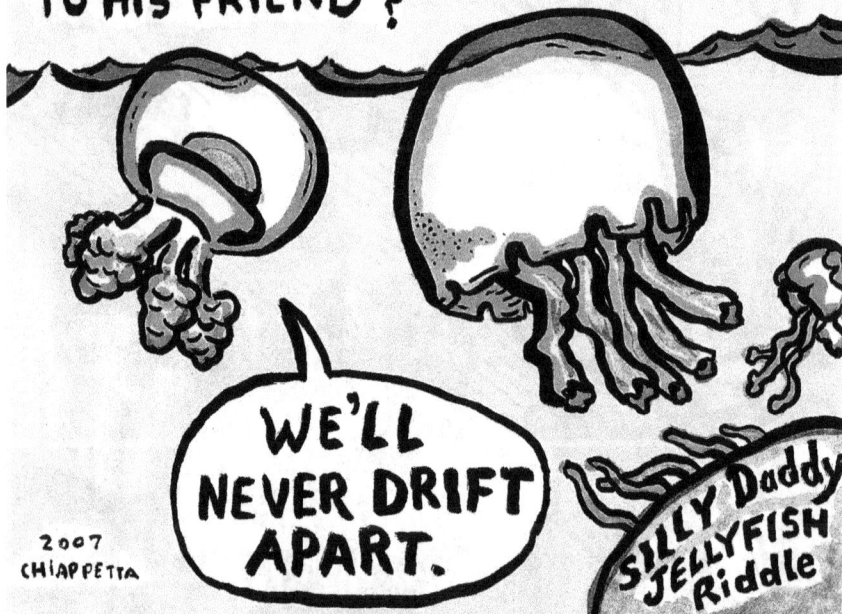

WHAT DID THE LOYAL JELLYFISH SAY TO HIS FRIEND?

WE'LL NEVER DRIFT APART.

2007
CHIAPPETTA

SILLY Daddy JELLYFISH Riddle

A loyal friend and good direction are worth their weight in gold, and they were exactly what I needed to get me through the next phase of my life. My own strength simply would not cut it anymore.

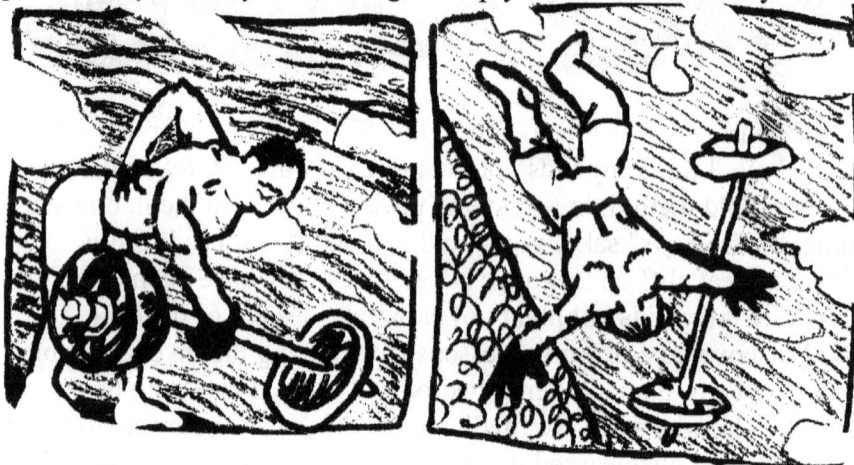

Chapter 4:

How Many Disabilities Do I Really Got?

There are so many great songs about loyalty. Growing up in the Chicago suburbs, I recall a song by Sonny and Cher that breaks my heart every time I hear it. The song "I've Got You Babe" is all about loyalty and reliance on each other. Listening to such a tune, you'd be certain that, as they took turns singing their parts, this couple could never be shaken apart. However, when you note the reality of the people behind the song--that they actually got divorced in real life-- it's quite tragic. Sonny and Cher don't have each other anymore. Conflict in their life tore them apart.

Whether it's relationship issues or disability issues, both come with conflict. I have found that the best way to rescue any situation involving conflict must involve prayer. My friend Roger, with his booming bass voice, says it best; "If you want to resolve conflict, begin with prayer." It sounds quite powerful coming from this old buddy of mine, not just because he walks the walk, but also because he looks like Moses.

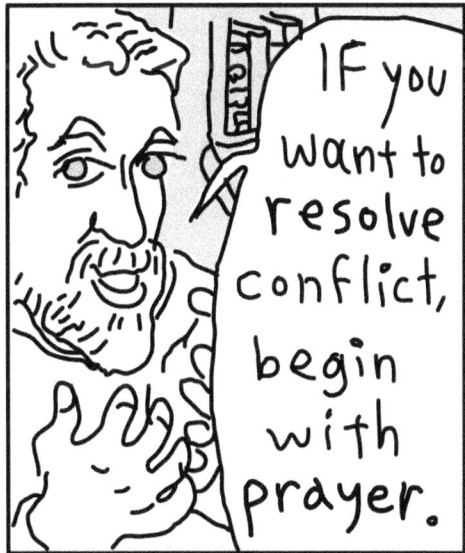

Sounding conflict-free, the Sonny and Cher song "I've Got You Babe" is still lovely many decades after it has been written. However, for those two singers, the song is simply not true anymore. The couple behind the tune was quite excellent at communicating the intense emotions that are bound up in a close relationship. Yet artistic statement of unfailing loyalty is not the same as actual loyalty. Until a relationship is tested, you don't really know what it is made of. The same can be said with the onset of a disability. It will test every relationship you have. With the rise of my own back injury, I have discovered that the more disruptive to life patterns that a disability becomes, the more that person's relationships get tested.

This is a hot topic for me, because I have lost relationships over disability issues, and current relationships can be strained and stretched in the process. Case in point, a few years ago, my wife Denise and I were having an argument at the Brookfield Zoo. I'm sure I was not on my best behavior due to the constant irritation and distraction of back pain, and I would often come across as tired or no fun.

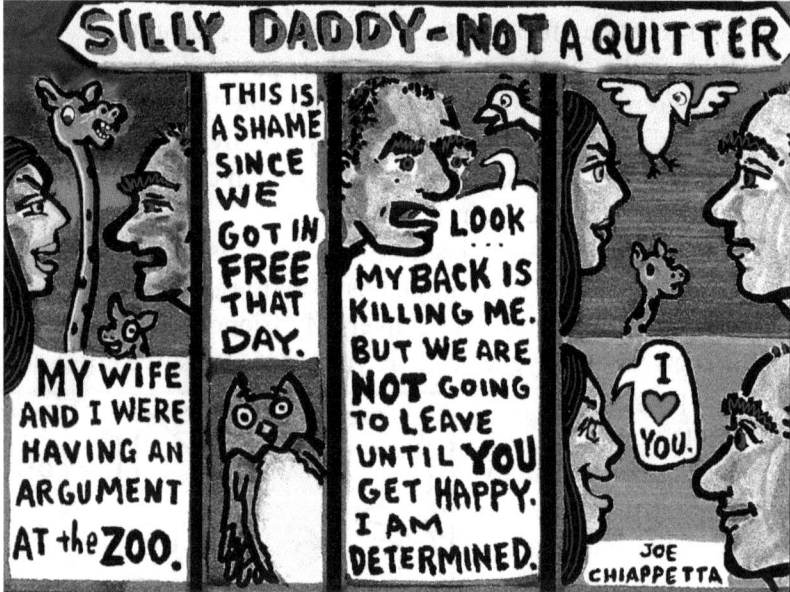

Just after our zoo argument was resolved, Denise said, "You have to do a comic about this." Here we have a true story about how zoological romance almost got derailed by my disability. Denise loves to tell this story because our wild determination not to give up is the very element that makes our marriage so resilient.

Admitting that my reaction to chronic pain has often been a hindrance in my marriage is completely uncomfortable and embarrassing. Emotionally, it's safer to look at disability from the perspective of two tulips. What's not to like about tulips? They are one of the first flowers to bloom in the spring, and they resurrect the next year. But these fine flowers are not without their problems, especially seen from the eyes of a man in the throes of his own back spasms.

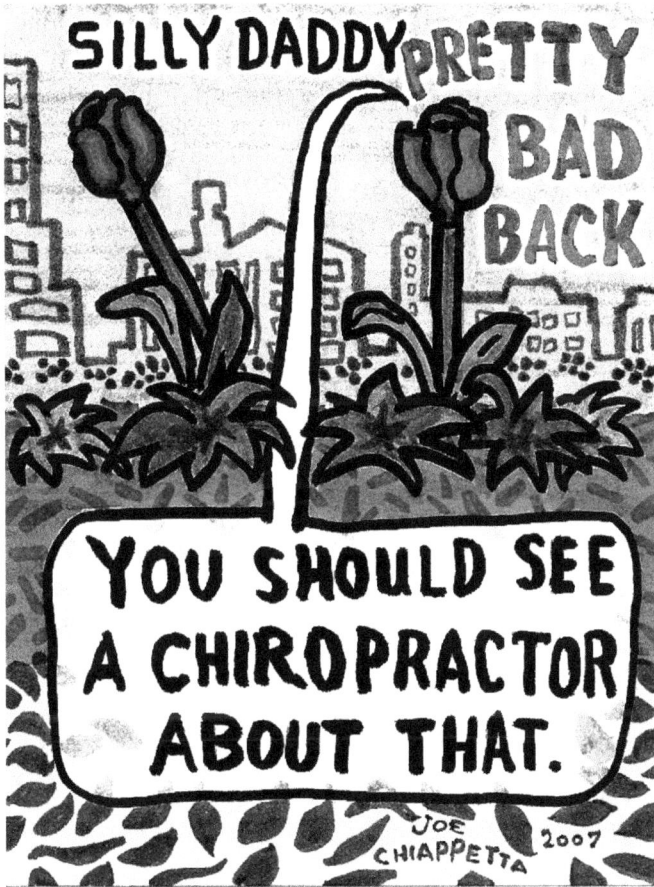

Multiple people have suggested that I see a chiropractor over the years. But only a handful would go that extra mile, come to my house, and pick me up so I could lay in their back seat pain-free while they drove me to where I needed to be. You see, my injury wouldn't allow me to sit for more than a few minutes without extreme discomfort. Those few who opened their back car seat to me are my real friends. As Sonny and Cher sang with such passion, **"I got you, won't let go... I got you to understand!"** Moreover, my true friends not only sing it, but they also live it. That's loyalty. They've "got" me, babe.

If only I could sit without pain and not be such a burden to these good friends and family members. I remember watching an old science fiction TV show wherein the main spaceship on the show had a unique control area that I thought was so awesome, I wanted it. The way their pilots had to drive the ship was to lie on their stomach to access the controls. Surely it looked bizarre to the rest of the viewing public. But to me, it was brilliant. That was the future!

Thereafter, it became routine for me while driving alone and thinking about how my back was killing me to ask, "Why can't they make cars where you drive while standing up or lying down? Maybe I should start a company that does so."

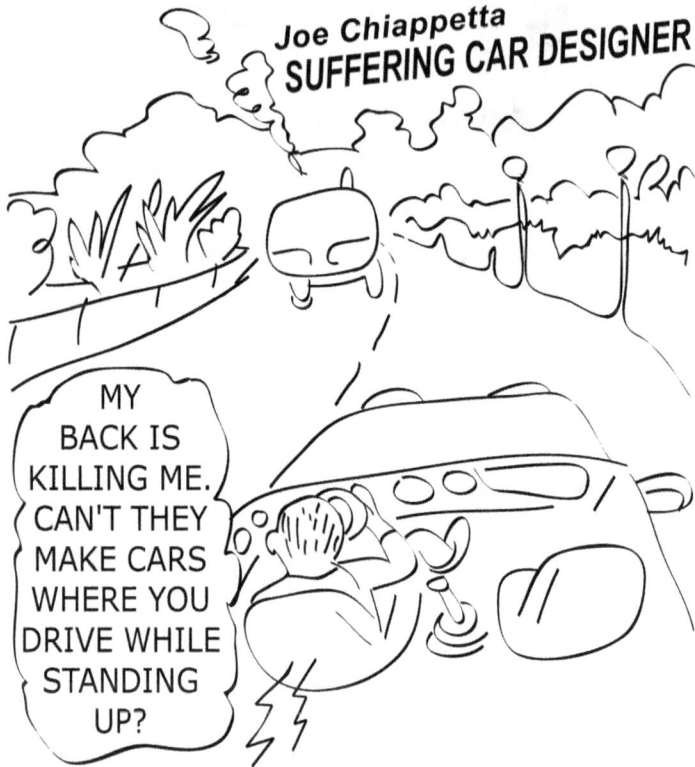

I don't know what I would have done without the loyal people in my life who picked up the slack for me while I waited in vain for the invention of cars a man could drive from a standing position. Those friends gave me priceless genuine support. Denise, Lee, Roger, Dave, and Jay surely have a reward waiting for them in heaven.

Conversely, I believe pretended allegiance is one of the reasons that social networking sites like Facebook and Twitter have become popular. You can have the illusion of friendships, but the reality is that while these virtual connections appear as lovely as Sonny and Cher, they likely carry no more depth of loyalty than that of a tragically divorced couple.

With the growth of Internet social networking, shallow contacts with fake loyalty will only increase, as will the number of people putting their security in how many online connections they have. For those who use social networking sites like Facebook, Twitter, Myspace, LinkedIn, Google Plus, you know what I mean.

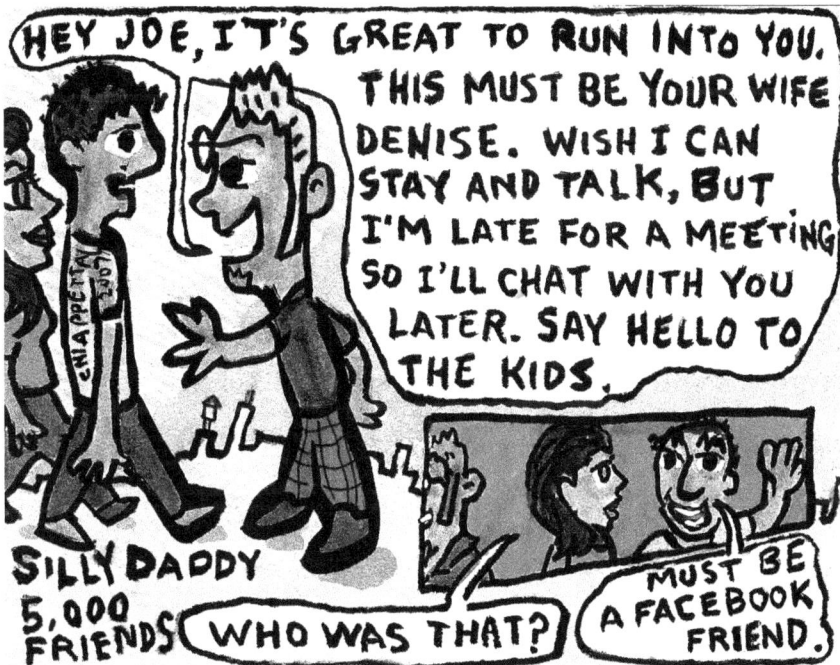

Incidentally, I once read that 5,000 was the limit to the number of "friends" a user can have on Facebook. I'm not sure if that is still the limit, but most people can't even manage five relationships well, let alone 5,000. Social media may be good for marketing, business networking, research, and lazy mode, but it is nowhere near replacing the types of relationships that give life deeper meaning.

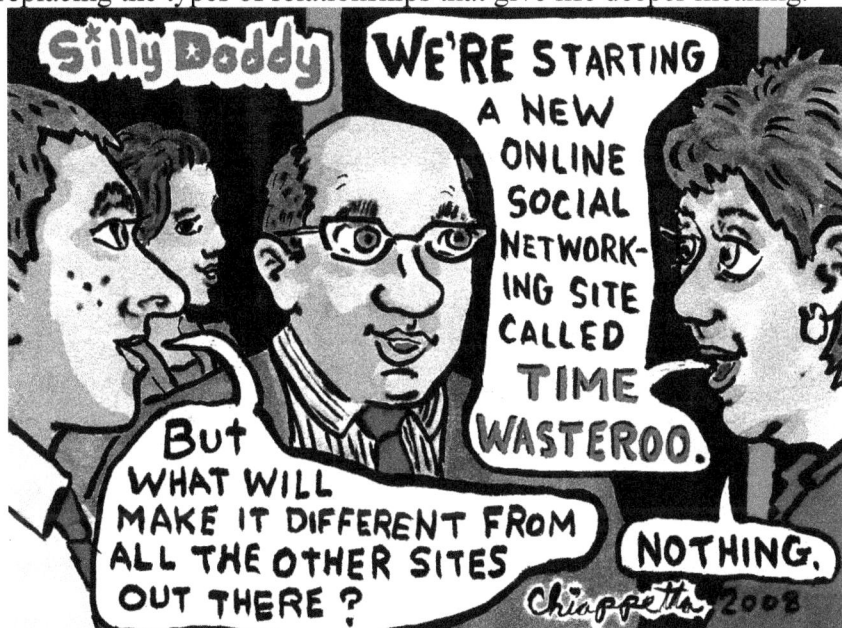

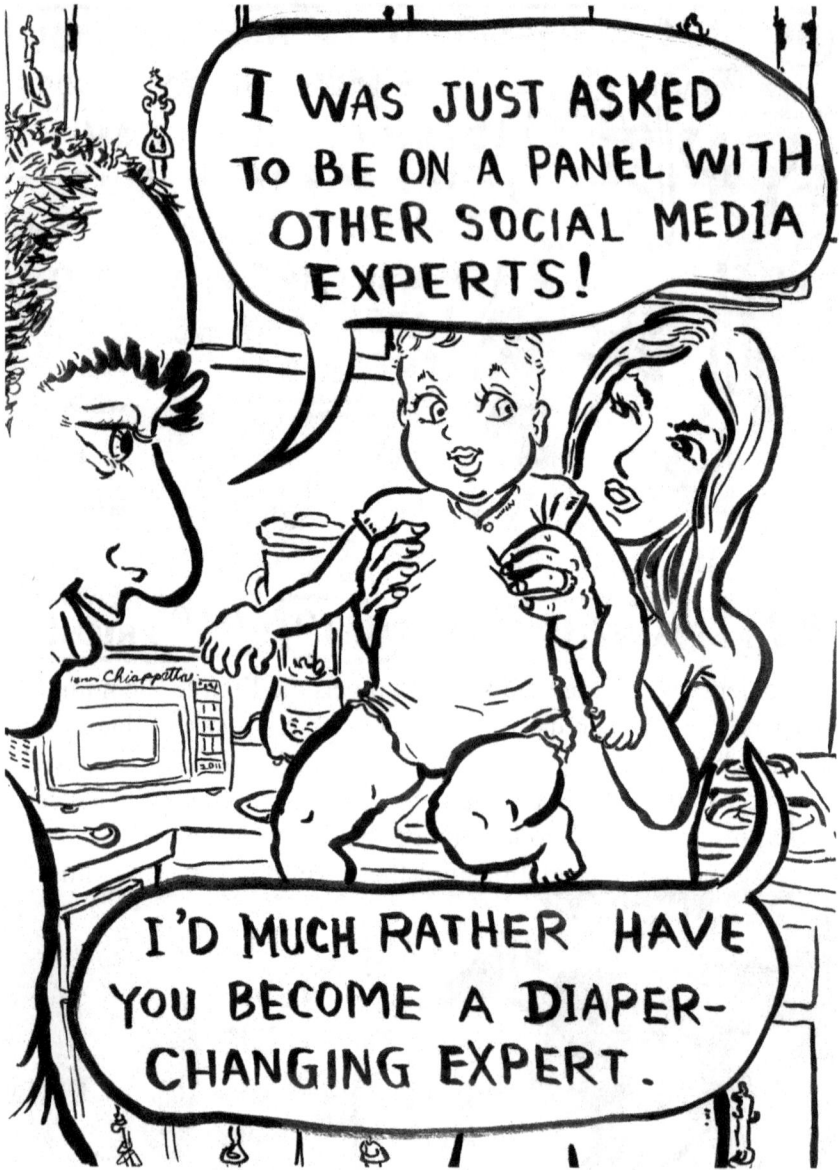

What else do loyal friendships have to do with disability? Everything. As your needs shift and even increase, you'll not only find out who your real friends are, but you'll also be able to inspire them by your perseverance. If you're not a quitter, they can learn from you, and if you are humble, you can learn from them. Make the most of the hard times.

I have good friends like Roger and my wife to remind me that humility is the key to everything. God knows that, but so often I forget it. Isn't that why, in his wisdom, God allows us to stumble through the challenges of this world?

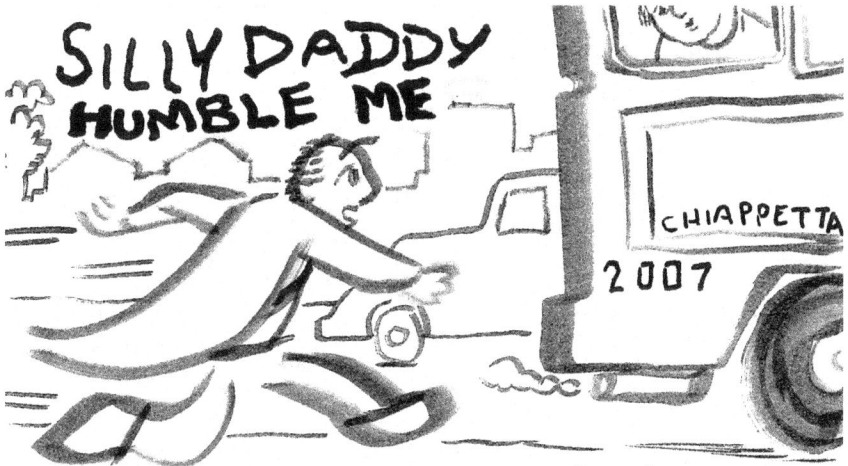

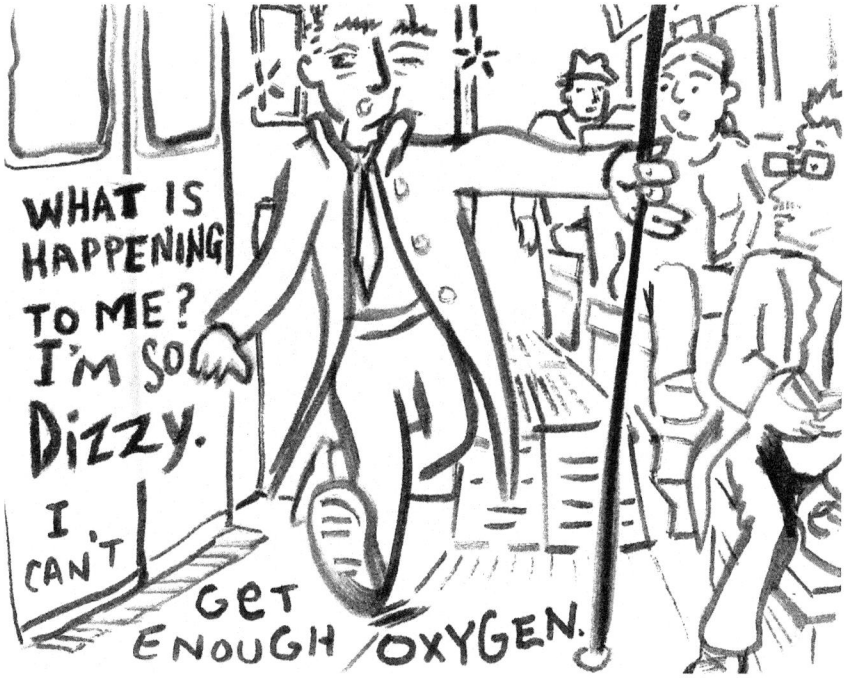

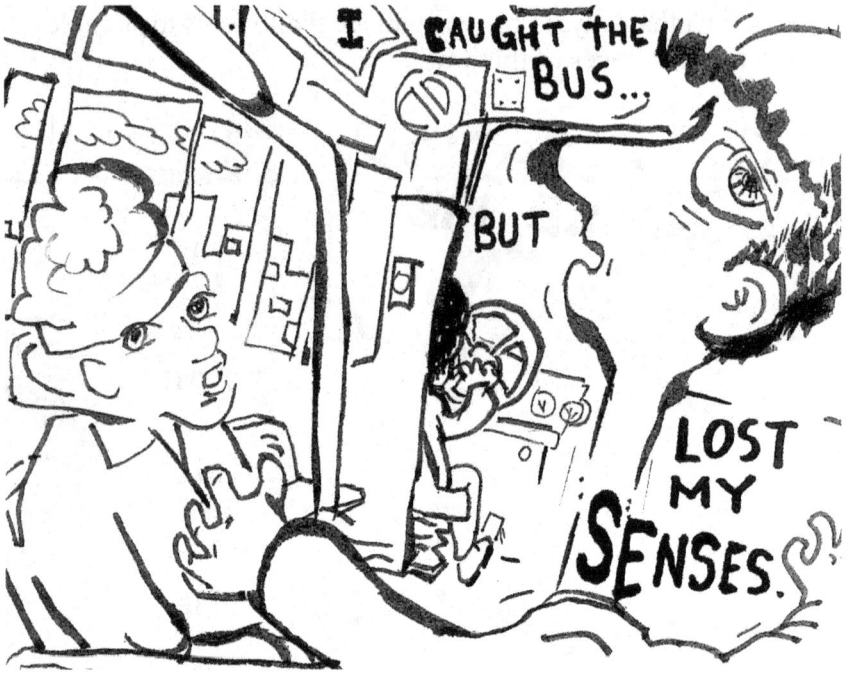

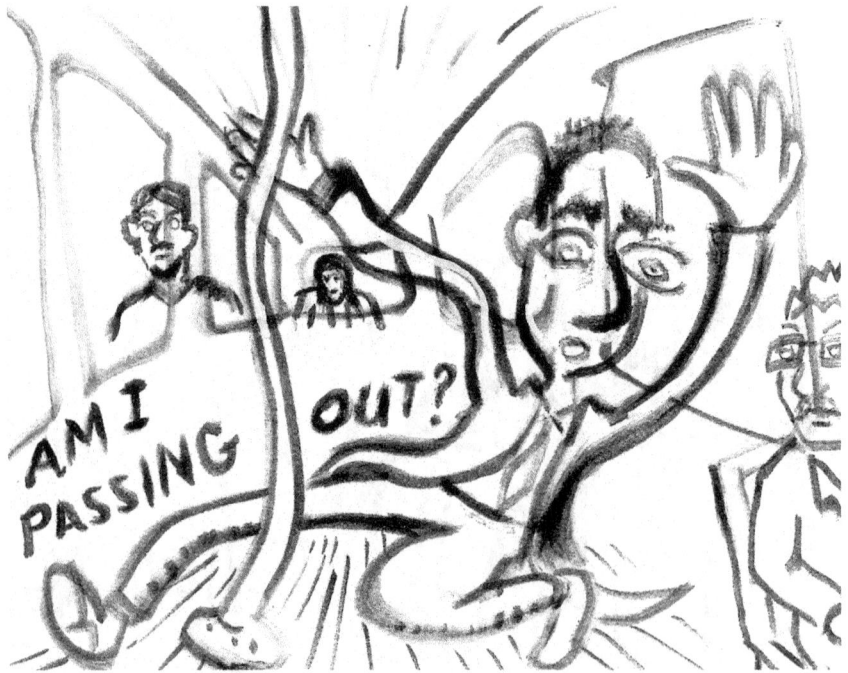

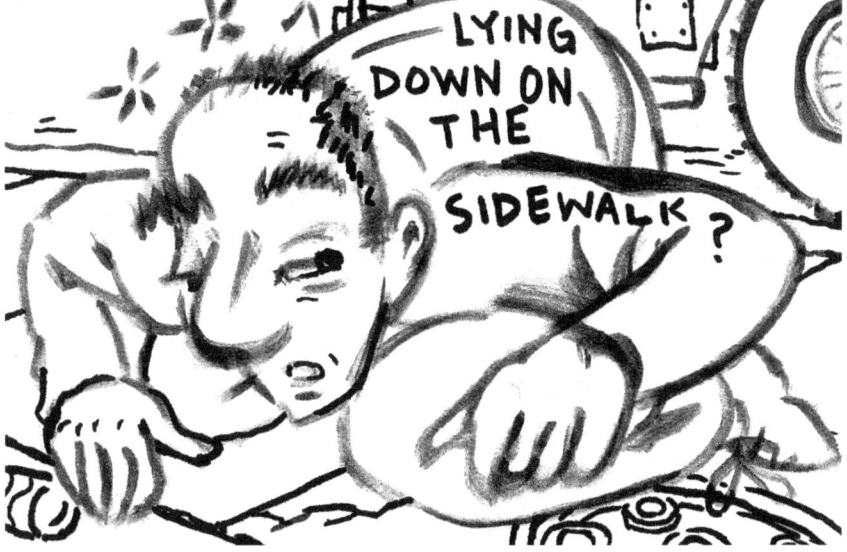

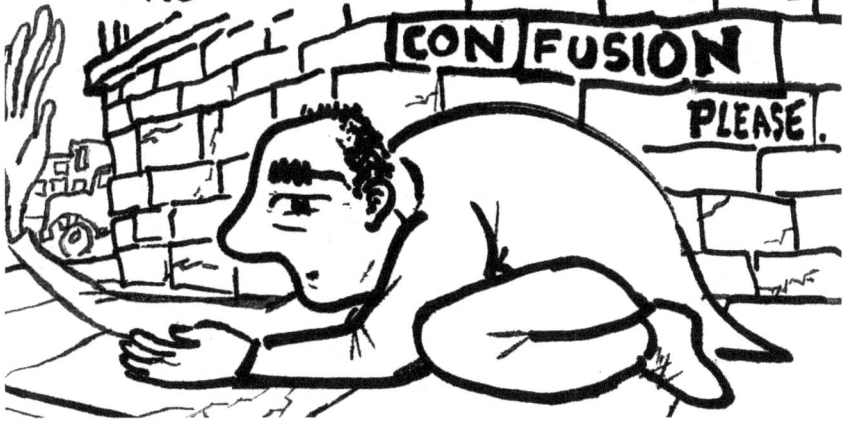

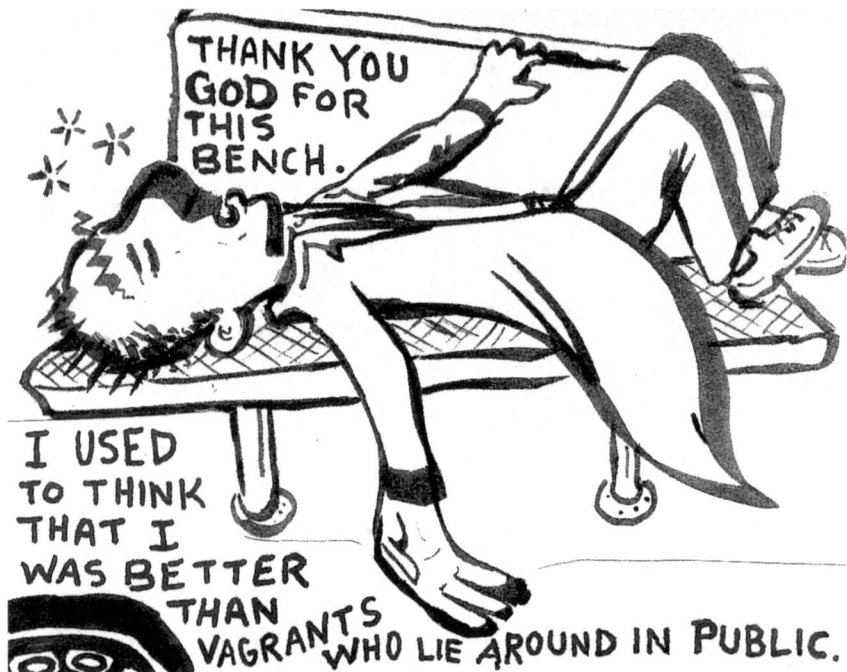

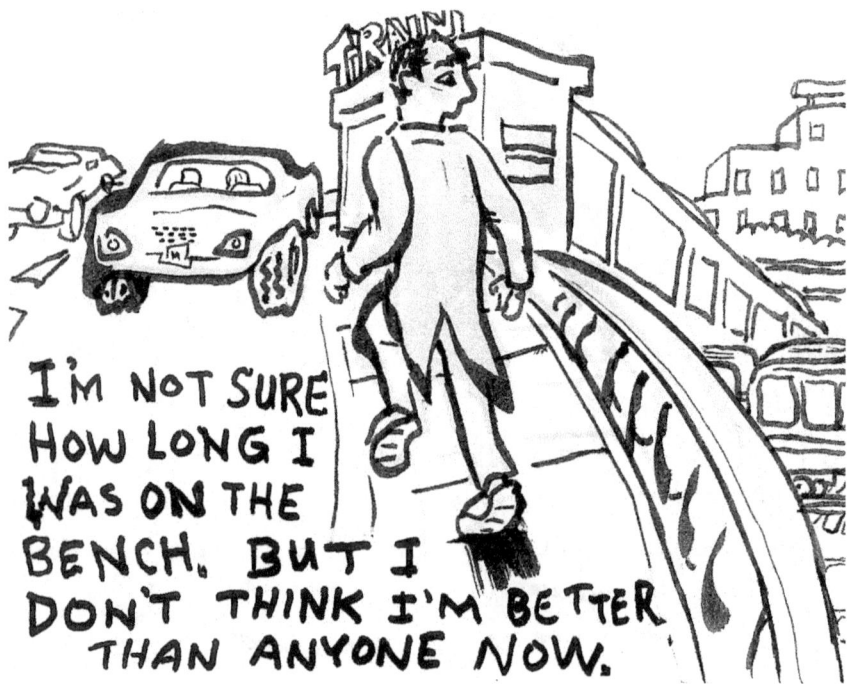

With this whole dizzy bus-chasing incident, God was doing something beautiful and even poetic with me. I chased with all my heart to catch a bus, yet will I do the same for God? Will I seek God with all my heart? Will I trust him even when all else seems to be eroding away, or am I fool enough to think that I'm strong enough to stand without the help of my God?

Psalm 18:27 explains God's attitude toward the humble and the prideful; it's even a salvation issue, so we all must get this concept down.

"You save the humble but bring low those whose eyes are haughty."

Since the word "psalm" literally means "song or poem," it seemed only fitting for me to reflect upon God's word and sing visually of the wise plan of God to humble me. At their best, that is what my comics can do: represent how God has brought me low and then saved me in my repentance and quest for humility.

Drawing upon another musical allusion, in the 1970s I had a favorite band and tried to memorize all of their songs. The Who, a British rock and roll band, sang a moving song called *How Many Friends Have I Really Got?* Talk about hitting the nail right on the head, the lyrics went on to explain the realities of relationships:

"You can count them all on one hand. How many friends have I really got, that love me, that want me, that will take me as I am?"

Much later in life, when I realized that I had multiple disabilities, the song became super profound. People typically treat you differently when you have a disability. They often feel weird, sad, or at the very least, unsure what they should say to a person with a disability--as if we speak an alien language.

But we don't. So just treat the person with a disability respectfully, as you would any other person, even if you can't be as helpful as you'd like to be.

Another time when I was traveling on the bus going from my house to Chicago, I helplessly observed a hair-raising scene that caused me to fear the declining course of my health. No harm came to me, but it was as if I were peering into the mirror of a possible future. The occasion involved an elderly man who used a motorized wheelchair. What I recall most about this man was the humility in his voice.

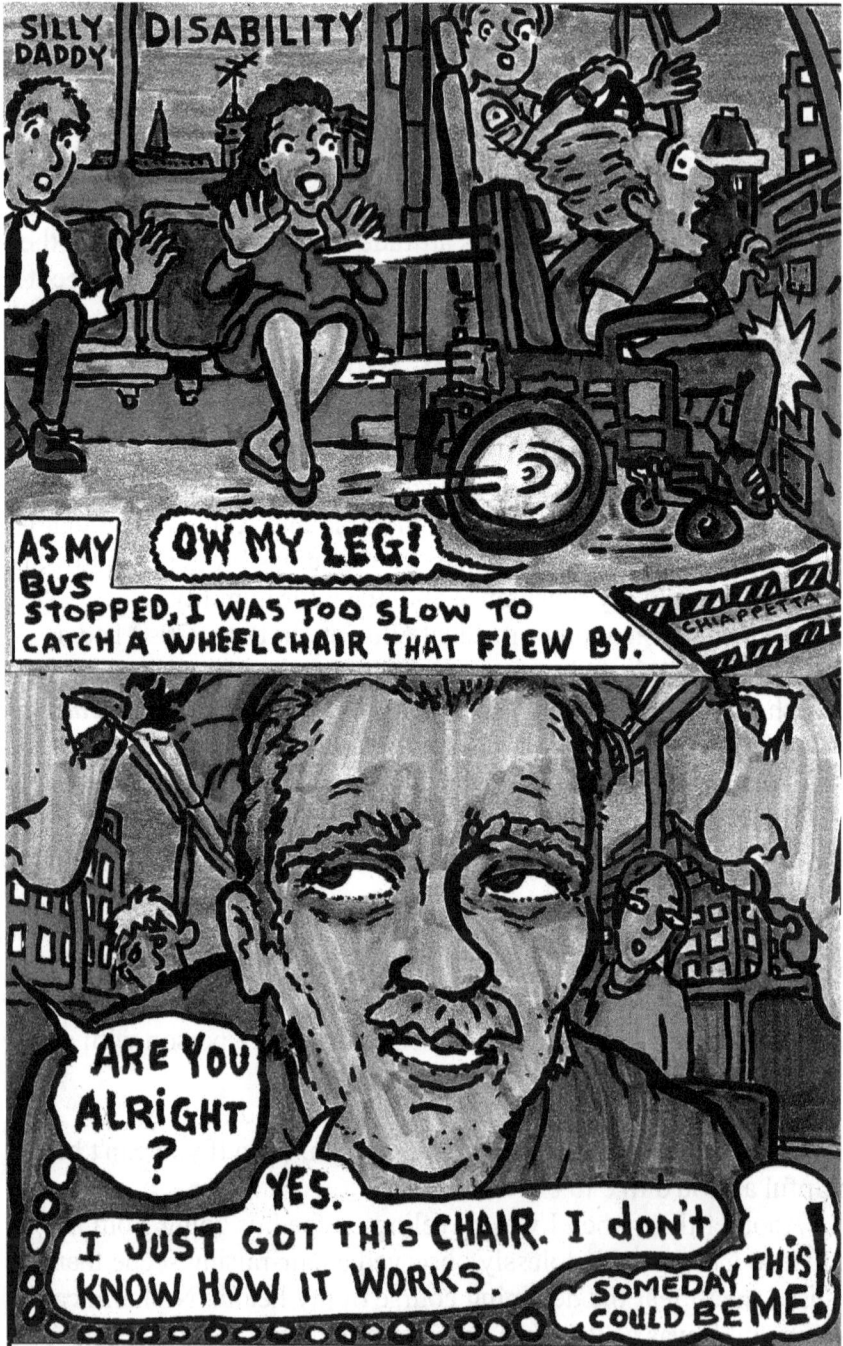

After the rolling wheelchair incident, what gave me some consolation while shoring up my own impairments was the positive attitudes of other people with disabilities I have known. Some of them I had merely heard in motivational speeches, like the fellow who addressed an employer breakfast once and gave the whole audience words to live by, including not quitting on life just because most of the world is oblivious to your struggles.

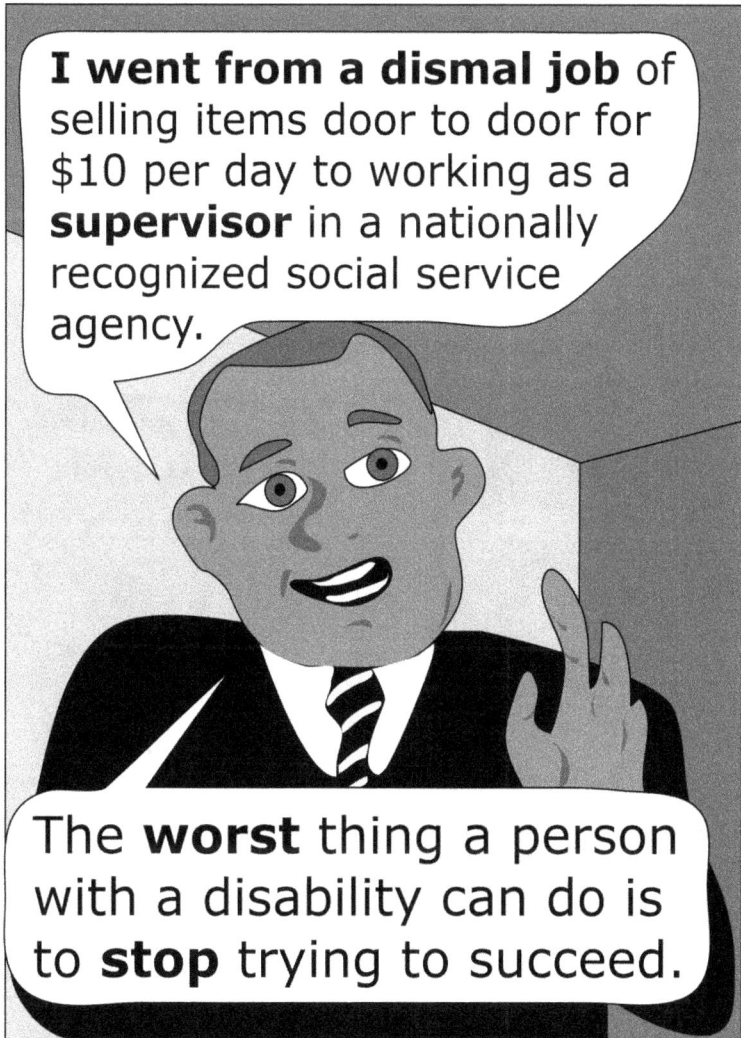

A good number of friends I've made have been people who use wheelchairs, and most of them can speak up a storm as well. Some talk openly about their disability, and some don't. It's their choice.

One particular friend of mine, Pat, has had a spinal cord injury for as long as I have known him and uses a wheelchair. Yet he has a can-do approach to challenges that would inspire anyone. Sure he has a disability, but so what! He also has confidence--heaps of it. I will never forget a conversation I had with him when we first met. The man was a tiger on wheels.

I know he was imitating Marlon Brando from some old movie, but the way he said this--his mannerisms and secure tone of voice--instantly told me that this person believes in his ability to sell me just about anything. That's an incredible skill to have.

Despite the fact that technically, I had to look down toward Pat in order to have a conversation, he clearly stands out as someone to look up to. I even remember thinking, "Worst case scenario, if my back gets worse and I do end up like Pat, at least I have someone to imitate."

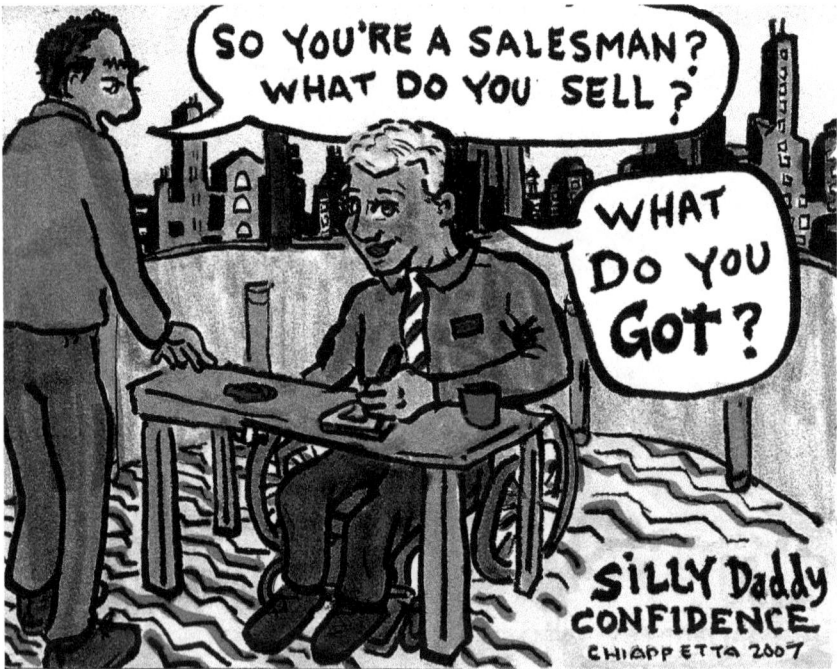

SO YOU'RE A SALESMAN? WHAT DO YOU SELL?

WHAT DO YOU GOT?

SILLY Daddy CONFIDENCE
CHIAPPETTA 2007

Chapter 5:

Accommodations I Have Known

What do the following have in common: a freezer, empty boxes, kneeling, the floor, and a house? Applied creatively, they kept me from getting fired by my employer because of a disability. Used the right way, these elements all had something to do with the work accommodations I made that allowed me to continue doing the essential functions of my office job. Keeping a job while having the very worst episodes of back pain can be very challenging, to say the least.

Over the years, I have implemented a number of workplace modifications to reduce the flare-ups of back pain. In the world of employment law, these are called "reasonable accommodations for workers with disabilities." Some of the job accommodations I have made are obvious, yet for the purpose of leaving no spine unturned, it might be useful to mention these on-the-job accommodations in more detail.

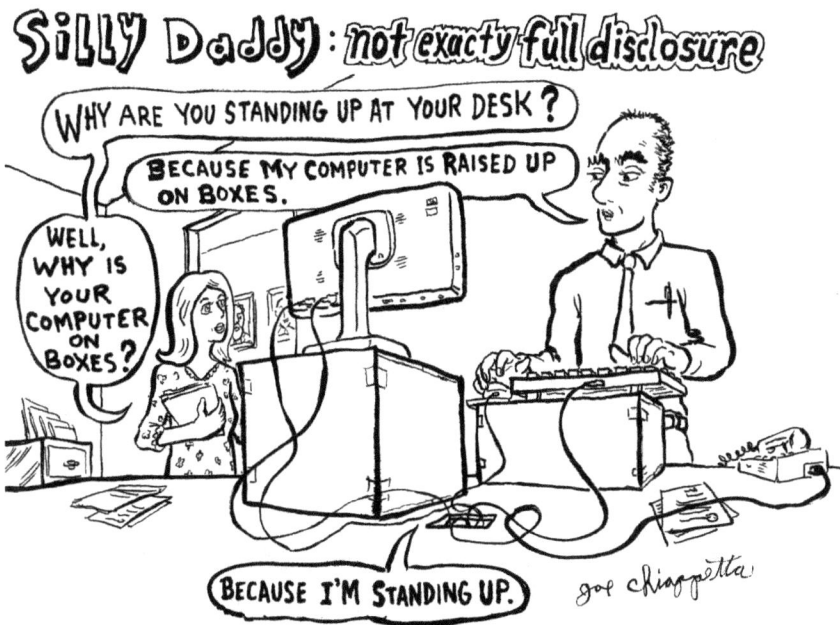

Silly Daddy: not exactly full disclosure

WHY ARE YOU STANDING UP AT YOUR DESK?

BECAUSE MY COMPUTER IS RAISED UP ON BOXES.

WELL, WHY IS YOUR COMPUTER ON BOXES?

BECAUSE I'M STANDING UP.

joe chiappetta

All in the name of adapting so I could still do my job, I would stand up at my desk rather than sit because my lower back pain, while in a seated position, was often unbearable. Therefore, I got a box, put my monitor on it and also put my keyboard on a box too. While this redecoration never made for the prettiest office, raising my work station was a no-cost way for me to ease my back pain, since sitting down was often like kryptonite for me. There's no accommodation like a corrugated cardboard accommodation.

Coworkers would often ask about this unique office setup. Sometimes I would explain why I reconfigured my workstation. Yet other times, especially when I didn't want to deal with my health issues, I would not take the time to clarify much of anything because I didn't want to disclose my disability to every passerby.

While raising or lowering a workstation to accommodate a disability on the job might be considered a best practice, talking in the evasive or abrupt manner in which I did in this conversation might fall more into the "worst practices" category. The world needs more people with disabilities to clearly, consistently, and patiently communicate the importance of disability awareness in everyday society.

Ice packs, not to be confused with Italian ice, were also very helpful on the job. My employer let me use the freezer to keep my ice packs cold, and I would put an ice pack on for 15 minutes at a time, about once an hour. This was an instant and drug-free way to relieve pain, and I couldn't have made it through the work day without those ice packs. Most pain medications give me bad side effects, so I am a big fan of the ice pack.

While kneeling during a meeting is a little unusual, I also practiced this frequently to reduce the stress on my back from sitting. Whenever people would ask about it, I would resist the urge to tell them that I was praying continually, like the Bible states. Rather, I often stated the simple truth; "My back is messed up and sitting hurts." That said, I sure wore out the knees on corduroy pants a lot quicker than the average office worker.

Not unlike explaining the boxes in my office, there were more than a few odd times where I was so frustrated with everything about my disability, that I would kneel at a meeting and not even attempt to explain my position. Those days I was fit to be tied, and it's unlikely that I would have been able to pass any sort of psychosocial behavior test. It was for occasions such as these that the phrase "You should have stayed in bed," was made.

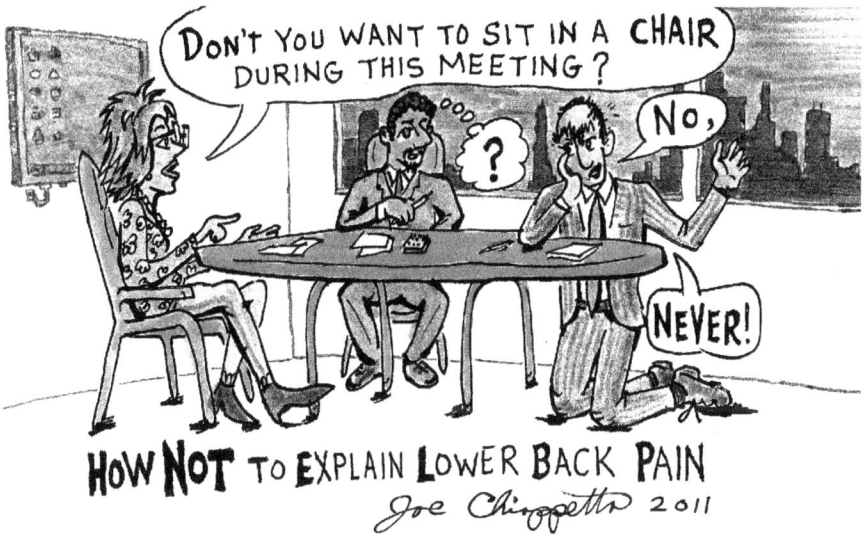

HOW NOT TO EXPLAIN LOWER BACK PAIN

Joe Chiappetta 2011

This, of course, is how **not** to explain lower back pain at the office, or probably anywhere else, for that matter.

Frustrations aside, I am grateful that for some of my work life, I've had the luxury of having an office with a door. Therefore, whenever possible, I would close the door and work while lying on the floor. No, I never fell asleep in such a position. In fact, I was often more productive because I was not distracted by pain. Drafting reports, making phone calls, attending webinars and conference calls could all be done just as effectively from the floor lying on my stomach or back.

Working from the floor, of course, was even easier to do when my employer started letting me work from home. Slowly but surely, more and more companies are adopting telecommuting as a viable option for responsible workers--also known as "telework." This will increase as companies continue to shift from an attendance-based mentality to an outcome-based mentality. More and more in the future, companies won't care where or how the work gets done, as long as it gets done cheaply, efficiently, legally, and with high quality. Some people label working from home under the banner of "work/life balance." Personally, I am pushing for a new term, "pajama professionals," but that's just me.

It is quite remarkable how the business community is embracing work-from-home models more and more. Times sure have changed in this area. As telework eventually reaches full saturation among office employees, it could be one of the most significant changes in labor since the implementation of the forty-hour work week.

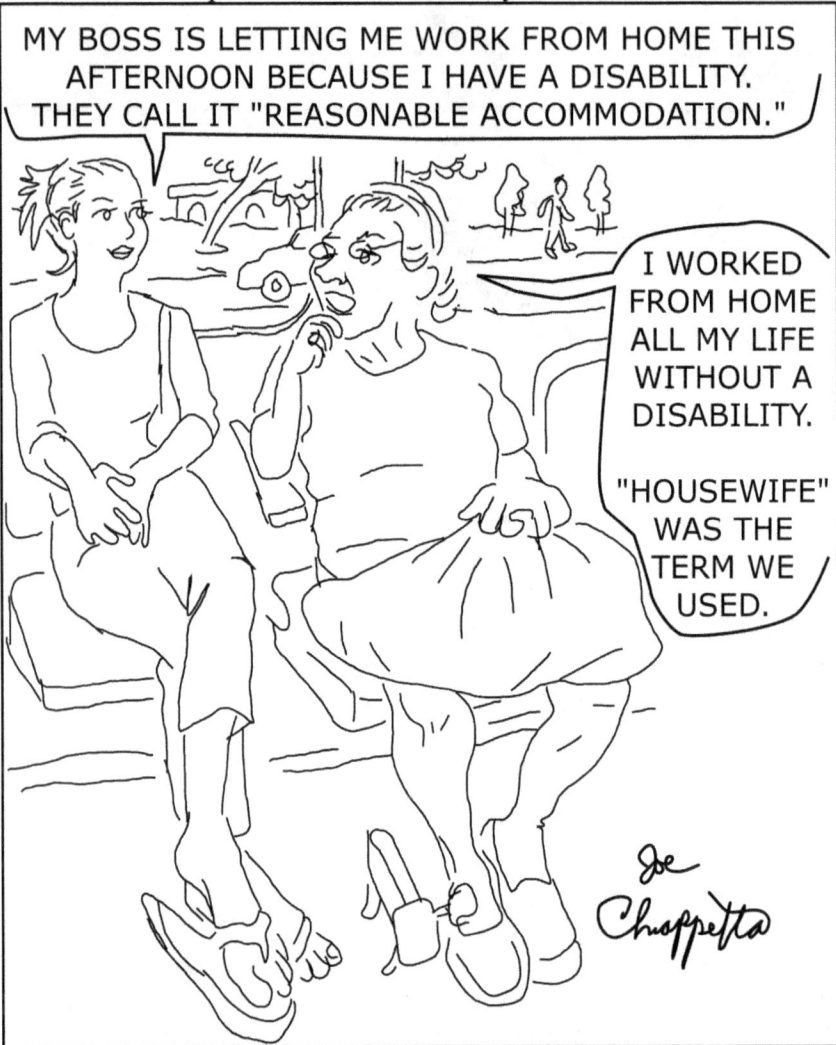

MY BOSS IS LETTING ME WORK FROM HOME THIS AFTERNOON BECAUSE I HAVE A DISABILITY. THEY CALL IT "REASONABLE ACCOMMODATION."

I WORKED FROM HOME ALL MY LIFE WITHOUT A DISABILITY.

"HOUSEWIFE" WAS THE TERM WE USED.

Embarrassing as it may be to admit, even while implementing all these accommodations, including telework, for much of my life, I would compare myself to people with apparent disabilities and not even consider myself as being disabled because my disabilities were usually non-apparent. While I was shoulder-deep in disability issues and heath impairments were shooting through my nerves, I was vehemently afraid of being classified and rejected by society. Who wants to be regarded as "handicapped," or "disabled?" Hardly anybody, that's who.

Chapter 6:

Fearful First and People First

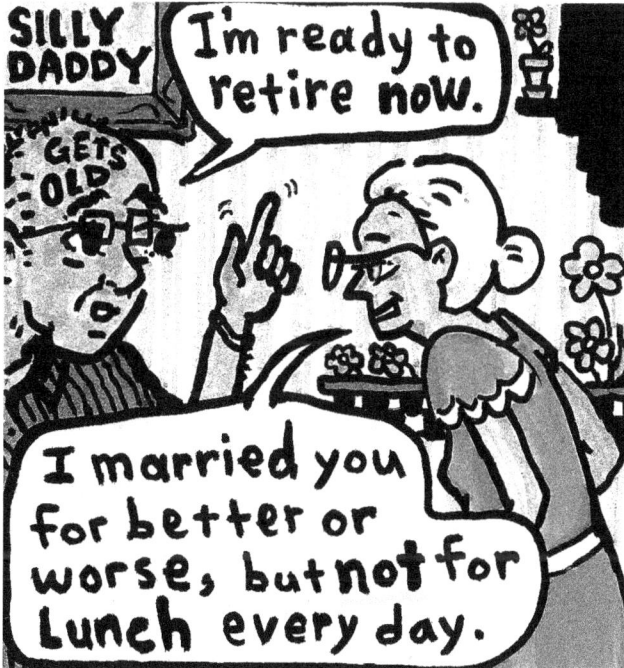

An examination of workforce patterns reveals a common theme among retirees; when one spouse retires while the other is already operating at home independently, for the first time (perhaps ever) the couple will be together more hours during the day (like for lunch). This can be a big adjustment for the spouse who previously had more time to herself in the middle of the day.

I feel compelled to highlight a number of points about the comic panel "Silly Daddy Gets Old," as there are a few wrinkles that need clarification.

1) The comic is not a real conversation that I've had. My wife really does like it when I can be home for lunch, as do I.

2) I am nowhere near retirement age.

3) On the surface, the comic seems merely like just plain fun. But there's a back story (pun not intended). The longer my chronic pain endured, the older I felt.

4) In fact, drawing myself thirty years older than I actually was came easy--too easy.

5) Growing concerns about how I would operate with a disability in such a discriminatory society increasingly seeped into much of my creative work and I was largely clueless about it.

Just look at a scene I drew in 1996, wherein *Silly Daddy* characters are stretching and aching after a long bus ride. This was not merely imaginative storytelling. That was how I felt every day. Yet there seemed to be no end to the aching and stretching.

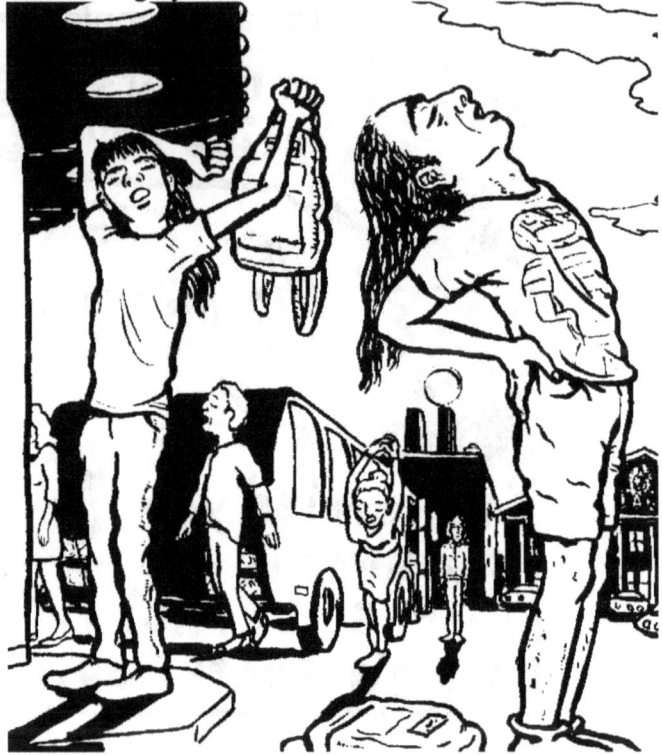

Disability concerns can even be seen in *Star Chosen*, my science fiction novel released in 2010. In the five years that it took to finish this book, I expressed a number of fears through a character named Darla Besto.

Darla is a CEO who acquired a serious mobility injury that landed her in the futuristic version of a wheelchair: a hoverchair. That's basically a chair with jets and anti-gravity features--the ultimate adaptive mobility device. Though my own situation never deemed it necessary, with the creation of Darla's hoverchair, I was mentally trying to prepare for the possibility of losing my ability to walk. That's how I dealt with it--self-imposed sci-fi art therapy. I realize now that the disability components of my stories were much more than creative impulses. Sci-fi disability themes were my coping mechanisms.

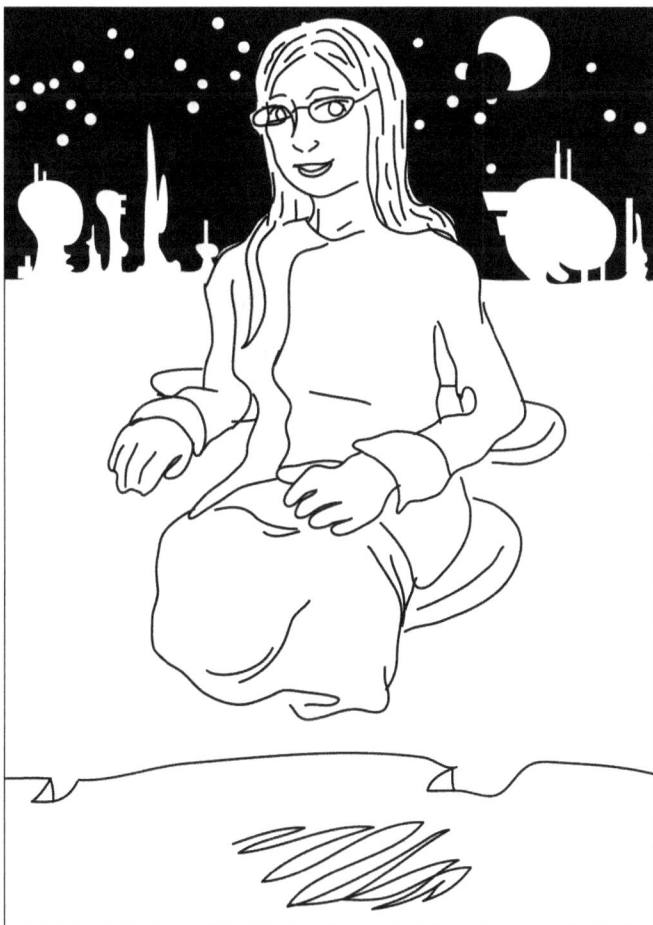

In one of the middle chapters of *Star Chosen*, Darla tried to explain some of her particular behaviors to a select few:

"You have to understand; for a person like me, with a disability, there is an even greater sense to prove myself. Why? Because the non-disabled population usually assumes I'm going to fail or come up short in life. They don't focus on my abilities, but only on my disabilities. And so it takes a lot to overcome that stereotype."

I never intended this, but looking back, I see that breaking through disability stereotypes is a significant secondary theme in *Star Chosen*. Another paragraph in the middle of the book hits this point head on. The narrator explains the views of a young teen named Tara regarding the larger-than-life Darla character:

"They were unpacking things and setting out blankets. Even Darla was helping. This was the first time that Tara recognized

that Darla was just a regular human being. Previously, Tara only identified Darla as 'celebrity,' or 'big Proud boss lady,' or even 'disabled overachiever.' Tara was embarrassed to admit that last label."

I've seen a number of people with disabilities, self included, adopt the attitude of "I'm an overachiever. Get used to it." On the surface, you might think that there's nothing wrong with talented people with disabilities highlighting their abilities. I'm not saying they shouldn't do so, but the very reason why it's so important to highlight abilities of people with disabilities is also the problem. People with disabilities often have to work harder and emphasize their abilities because many people's expectations plummet when the disability word enters the picture.

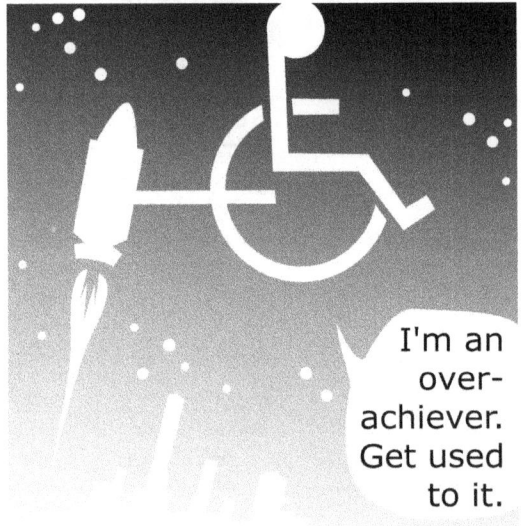

I'm an over-achiever. Get used to it.

I was barely conscious of it, but in retrospect, I used the Darla character as a major attempt to deal with a lot of my own health issues. Most readers wouldn't know this, however, because the book is loaded with all sorts of science fiction action. Nevertheless, earlier in that book, I wrote that Darla **"had one of her offices in zero gravity due to her disability. Of course she didn't spend a lot of time there, since zero gravity causes muscles and bones to weaken over prolonged periods."** That was really my own personal way of saying, "I really wish I could just lay on my back all day to rest and heal, but what if my muscles wither away in the process?"

Surprisingly, there are no less than three characters in the *Star Chosen* novel who have mobility or lower back issues. Take this scene from the first section of the book:

"In the dark of night, which is never really that dark in a city open around the clock, like Chicago, Tharquinn Thane slumped down to the ground. He pulled his mini back-rubbing machine out from his belt, and the device expanded to massage his aching back. From looking at him, a person would never guess that he had chronic back pain. He hadn't even hit middle age yet, and

his appearance was typically healthy and energetic. However, too many years of slouching, writing, and studying had a negative effect on his back. As a member of the minority class known as the Chosen, Tharquinn only recently became able to afford this expensive massaging device known as the iBaq..."

There's no denying the autobiographical nature of that segment. Yet, melodramatic sci-fi thoughts aside, not all of my disability ramblings were deep confessions of health-related anxiety. I fought to find a balance with light-hearted pieces as well.

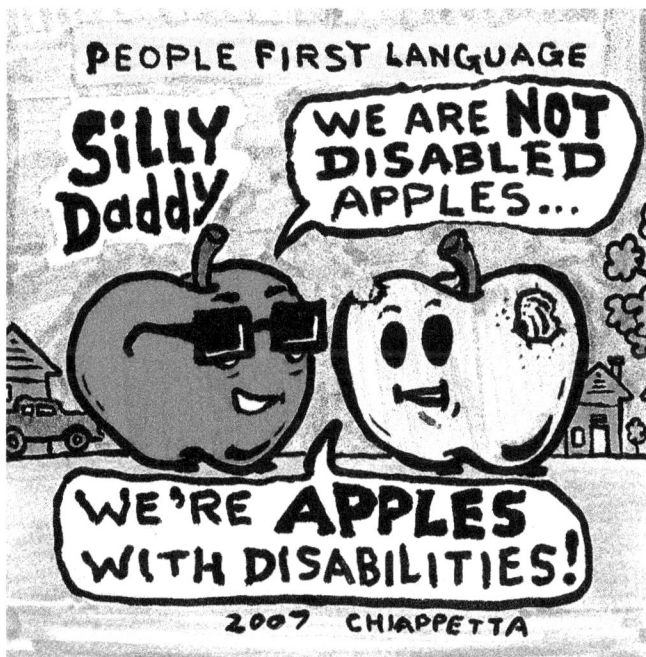

If you know anything about "people first language," my "apples with disabilities" comic is in sweet reference to the "people first" movement regarding disabilities. It is an effort to reduce the huge discrimination against people with disabilities in the world. Basically, the whole idea is not to label people as "disabled first." Rather, label all people as people first. The movement is aimed at not allowing a person's health condition to define who they are.

For example, when you have to talk about disability issues, rather than saying, "He's an autistic guy," it is preferable to say, "He's a person with autism." Here's another good example. Don't say, "She's a wheelchair-bound woman." Unless we're talking about some wild action movie plot where the hero is physically restrained in a chair by the diabolical villain, people are typically not bound (tied up) to any wheelchairs. Therefore, just say, "She's a person who uses a wheelchair," or even, "She's a science fiction character with a spinal cord injury." That would work in the *Star Chosen* universe.

Principles behind people first mentality have some parallels with a scripture from 1 Samuel 16:7. **"But the LORD said to Samuel, 'Do not consider his appearance or his height, for I have rejected him. The LORD does not look at the things people look at. People look at the outward appearance, but the LORD looks at the heart.'"**

From the time when Israel's future King David was about to be chosen, it is plain to see that God looks at what's in the heart, not at how a person appears outwardly. We need to imitate this attitude with all people, especially people with disabilities or physical differences.

Consider the plight of the oversized man known as Bigfoot:

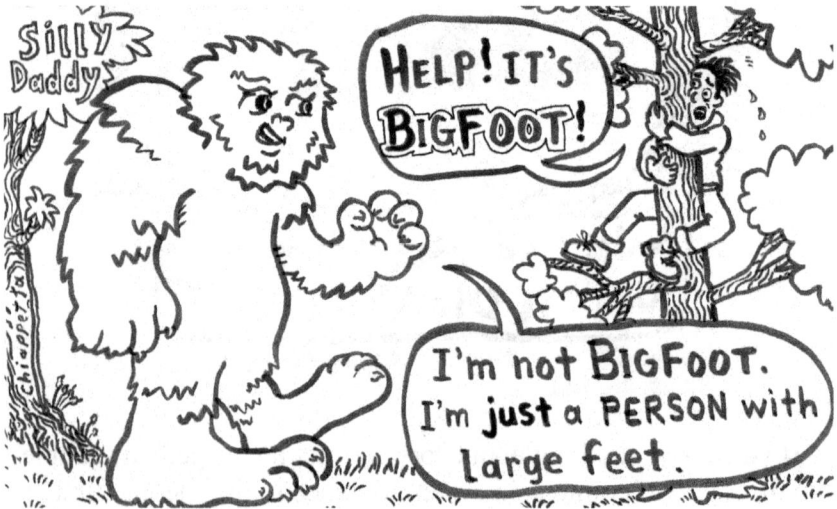

However odd a person might look, people have a basic desire to be regarded as people first. Nevertheless, the people first movement, while clearly defined, has not yet caught on in a widespread manner. It's not a mainstream household concept, and to the horror of hardcore disability advocates, perhaps it never will be. As such, I have observed much discriminatory behavior firsthand in life, as well as in my decade-long career helping other people with disabilities find jobs.

Words can be very powerful, and rethinking how we phrase disability concepts and terminology can go a long way in creating a culture of inclusion for people with disabilities. One friend of mine, Dave Stevens, pointed out how sometimes even well-intentioned places that serve people with disabilities can have names that send the wrong message. We only have a finite number of things to communicate before we die, so it is important to hit the target right on the first try. If such a thing is not possible, then it is best to change as soon as a better way to communicate comes to light.

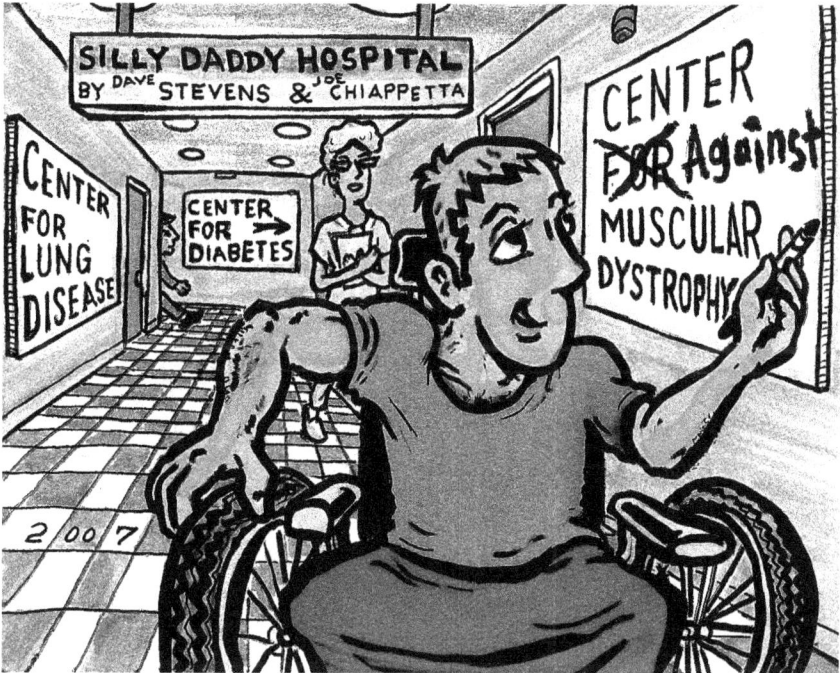

Dave Stevens is one of the many people I know who help people with disabilities find jobs. Victories do exist in the employment of people with disabilities, yet usually they are hard to come by. However, in a few rare cases, those employment victories seemed to happen with relative ease. The time I helped a would-be movie director comes to mind right away. I was working as an employment specialist helping people with developmental disabilities find jobs. Employed by a social service agency called Seguin, I was given free reign, as well as mileage reimbursement, to scour the earth in search of people and places open to the good news of hiring people with disabilities.

WOULD-BE MOVIE DIRECTOR'S SMASH HIT AT LIBRARY

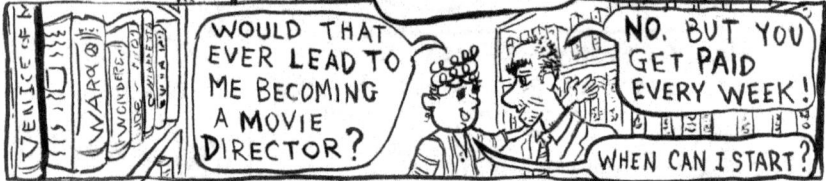

THE LIBRARY HIRED THAT JOB SEEKER, AND A DECADE LATER, HIS BOSS HAD THIS TO SAY;

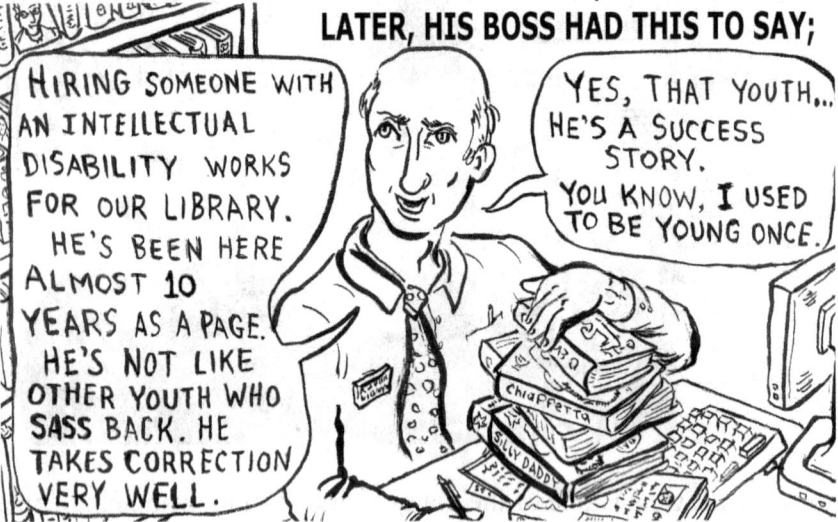

What I like so much about this success story is that we stayed as close as we could to the originally stated dream job of being a movie director. A dream job is what you would like to do if you could pick any job in the entire world, casting all barriers aside. Dream jobs, while often not ever achieved, are important to understand when helping someone find a job. Knowing where dreams and goals are pointing toward is helpful in finding out where those dreams and aspirations might be interested in settling along the way.

I have had a number of dream jobs over the years that never actually turned into real employment. Nevertheless, such interests do help us understand who we are, or at least who we want to be. For a while one dream job of mine involved exploring abandoned industrial areas wherein nature was starting to take over again. Something about the quiet remnant of bygone industry pitted against God's natural environment can be most fascinating for me. While I could never figure out how such an interest could lead to a paycheck, the hobby did bring me to a number of unique places and conversations, especially when I would bring the kids with me.

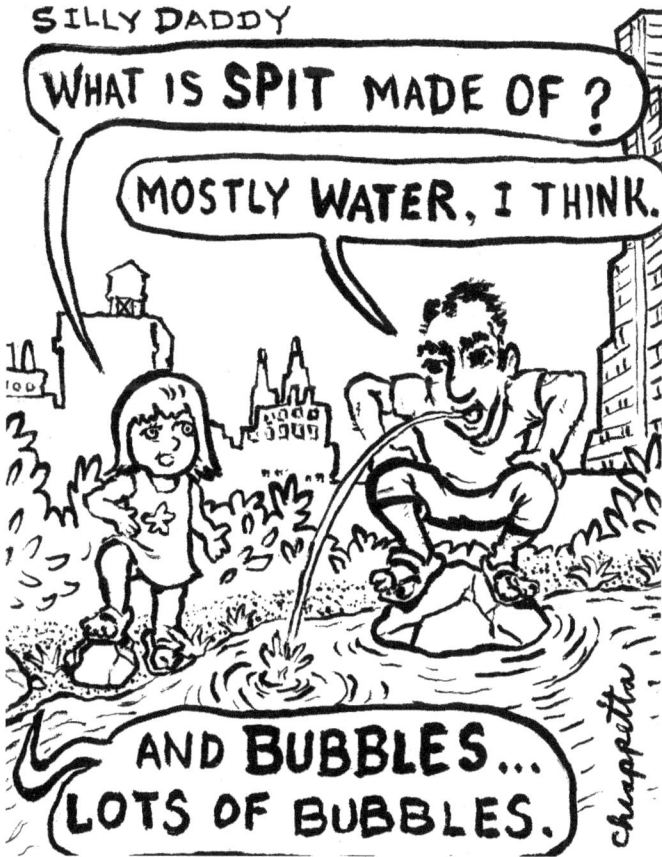

Once, after explaining what a dream job was to my son, it sparked an amusing conversation between siblings:

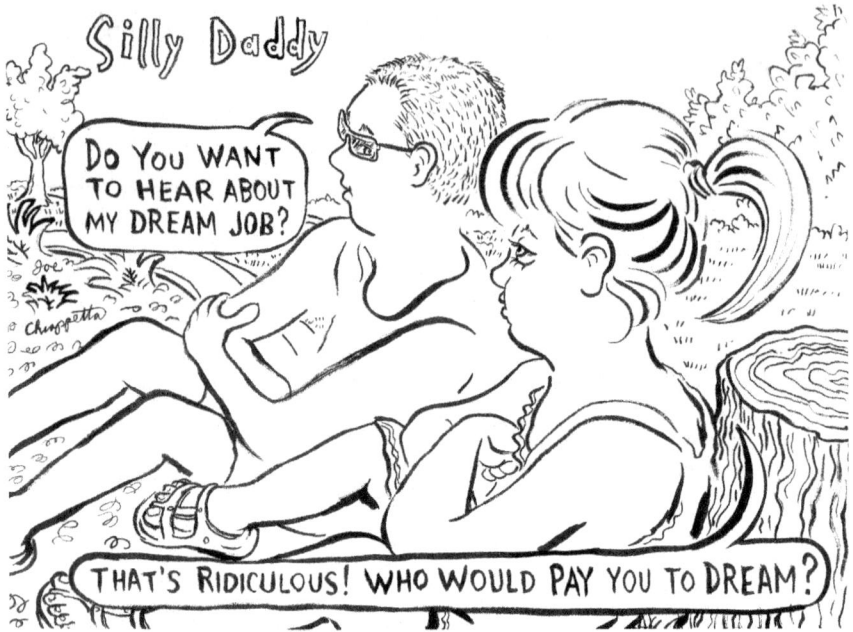

Silly Daddy

DO YOU WANT TO HEAR ABOUT MY DREAM JOB?

THAT'S RIDICULOUS! WHO WOULD PAY YOU TO DREAM?

Success stories and dream jobs aside, usually, when someone is labeled as "disabled," the false assumption people typically make is that the person with a disability won't be as useful, and could even be a problem to deal with. Dreams can be squashed right there in an instant decision. Because of these powerful stereotypes, I would often promote the hiring of people with disabilities as if I wasn't one of them. When I approached the library to get my client with the intellectual disability his job, the facts of my own disability were the furthest thing from my mind.

Nevertheless, from my teen years through my forties, I struggled with lower back pain as well as photo sensitivity, also known as light sensitivity. Both of these health issues have caused me to make modifications in my life that I would often take for granted. Yet as I grew older, these disabilities became more and more profound, and so did the modifications. For the light sensitivity, I increasingly have to wear sunglasses, even indoors, and rarely watch TV anymore--the light is just too bright. For the back pain, during the worst periods of it, just a few years ago, I couldn't even walk.

Despite the daily modifications I would make to function with these impairments, much reluctance and apprehension surrounded the thought of me actually talking about disability from a first-person point of view. I certainly could have, with medical professionals diagnosing me with a herniated disc, degenerative disc disease, early stage arthritis, bulging discs, the lifting restrictions, and the photo sensitivity. Whether I talked about these issues or not, I have come to realize that the longer a person lives, the more involved they will get in disability issues--like it or not. Eventually it will roll right into you. So I had to soberly ask myself, "How many disabilities do I really got," and how can I turn this into a strength?

I also learned who accepted me as a true friend during the worst symptoms of these disabilities. Just like the song, "How Many Friends Do I Really Got," I could count all my friends on one hand. I wouldn't have it any other way. I learned quite a bit from acquiring these disabilities and am glad to have been refined by the whole unpleasant experience of overcoming adversity.

The question now was whether or not I would use my talents to lead people with disabilities into a better position in this dark world. If I step up and defend this cause, then couldn't I make a big difference? Alternatively, doing nothing makes me part of the problem.

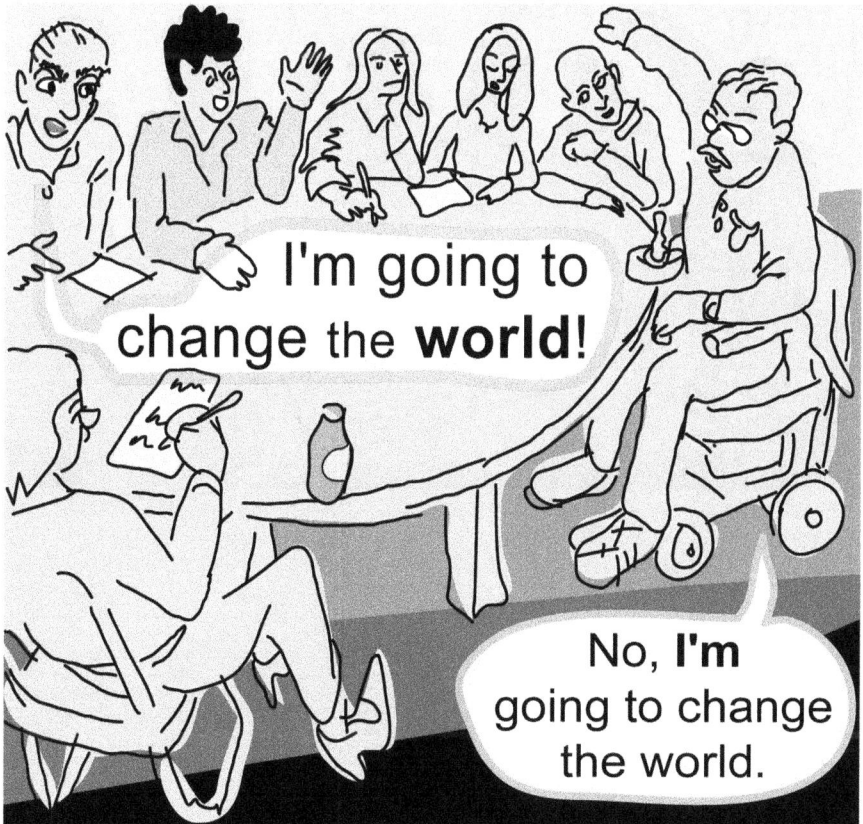

If I do set out to make things better, I must be prepared for opposition, even from those on my own side. I can see embarking on such an endeavor with a declaration that I am going to change the world! Care must be taken to guard against getting derailed by personality conflicts and fighting over funding.

Too often have I seen waves and waves of disability advocates (self included) wanting the same end goal, yet possessing selfish ambition, and being completely disunified about tactics and how to accomplish the end goal. Many get bogged down by minutiae, get distracted, and become inefficient in the cause. Consequently, little of significance gets done.

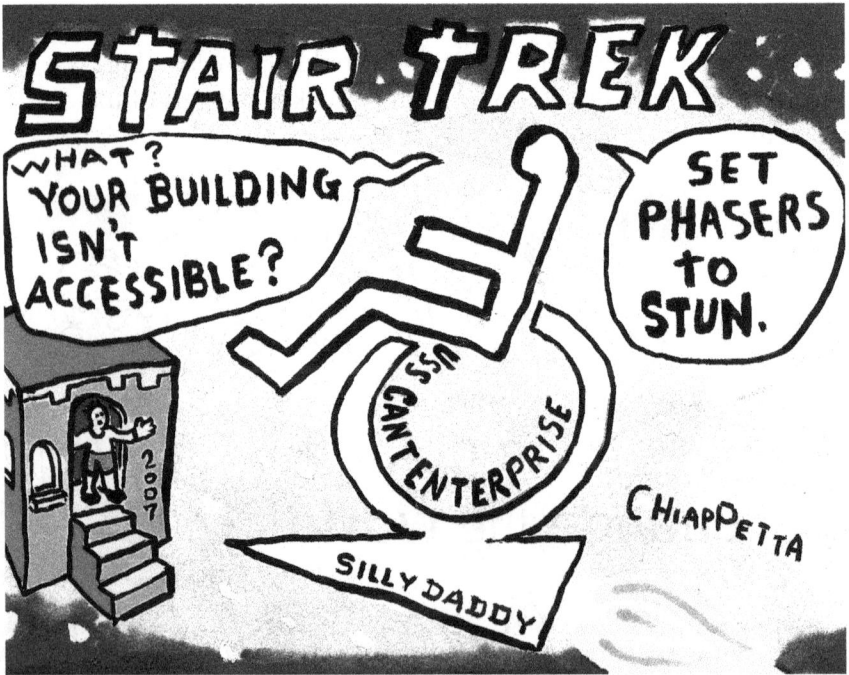

Chapter 7:

Disability Geekdom

While the desire to help others with similar impairments runs strong among many people with disabilities, heightened episodes of pain typically slow down goals toward that end. I know this firsthand.

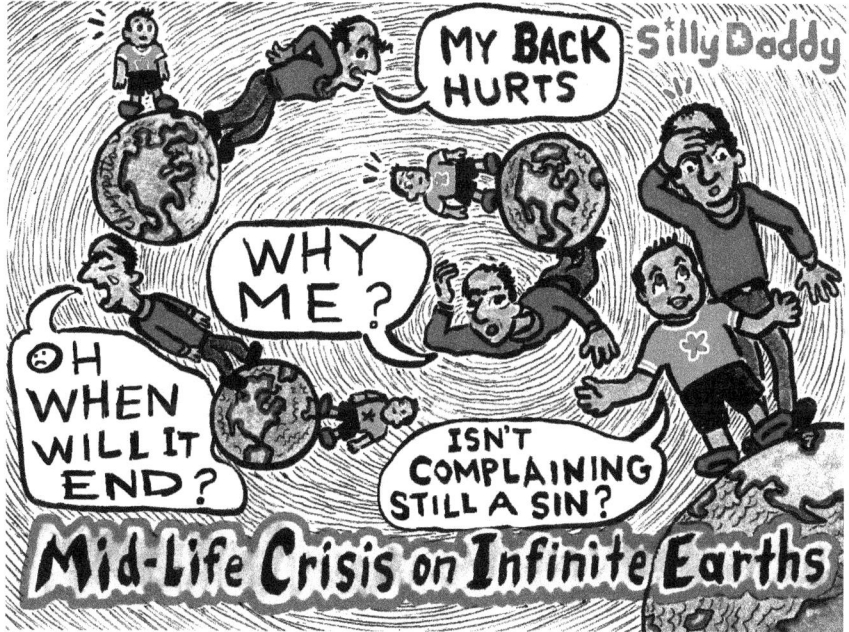

Since Philippians 2:14 says to **"Do everything without complaining,"** the answer to my son's stinging question is a solid "Yes." Nevertheless, while plagued by throbbing back spasms, it would still be difficult for me to picture anything but endless worlds wherein I grudgingly operated in constant distress.

Being raised on comic books, my imagination gravitated toward geeky scenarios that combined comic book themes with disability themes and became a creative outlet. Sometimes I felt like that was all I could do. My comic "Mid-life Crisis on Infinite Earths" is borrowing from a mainstream comic book called *Crisis on Infinite Earths*, published by DC Comics. I do realize that this pop culture reference is obscure and geeky, but no less obscure than many important disability issues. Thus do I enter into the halls of "Disability Geekdom."

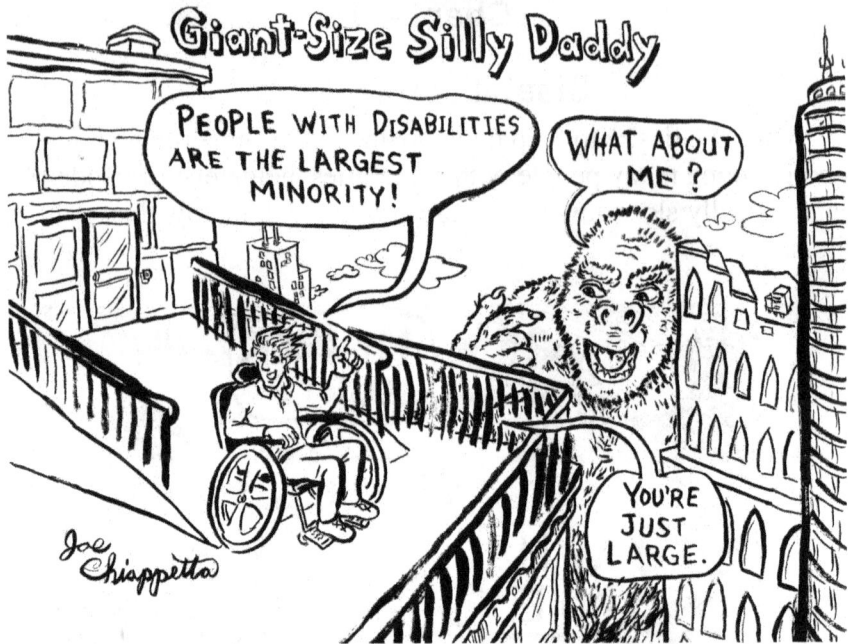

Giant-Size Silly Daddy

While giant monsters like King Kong, created by Merian C. Cooper, and Godzilla, created by Tomoyuki Tanaka, are fictional, it is quite true that people with disabilities are the largest minority in the United States of America. Like many fictional monsters, people with disabilities are often misunderstood and have a long history of being mistreated. Disability awareness, combined with brotherly love, can counter some of the unfair treatment that still exists in our society for people with disabilities.

One figure to emphasize is the amount of money that this group holds. A statistic from a 2002 US Census Bureau report puts the discretionary spending power of people with disabilities at over 200 billion dollars.

The numbers alone make a compelling case to pay more serious attention to this group. There are 54 million people in the USA who have a disability, according to the US Census Bureau (2005). That means one out of every five persons in the country is disabled. This is a significant number, highlighting that people with disabilities represent a rich diversity of individuals, and a major class of people to be thoughtful and respectful toward.

Moreover, in 2010, the World Health Organization said there were one billion people with disabilities on the planet. This is important to consider, showing that disability cuts across all races, continents, and countries. On a more personal level, it's likely that most people have a parent, sibling, friend or other family member that has or did have a disability. Taking into account accidents and sudden illnesses, disability can happen to anyone at any time.

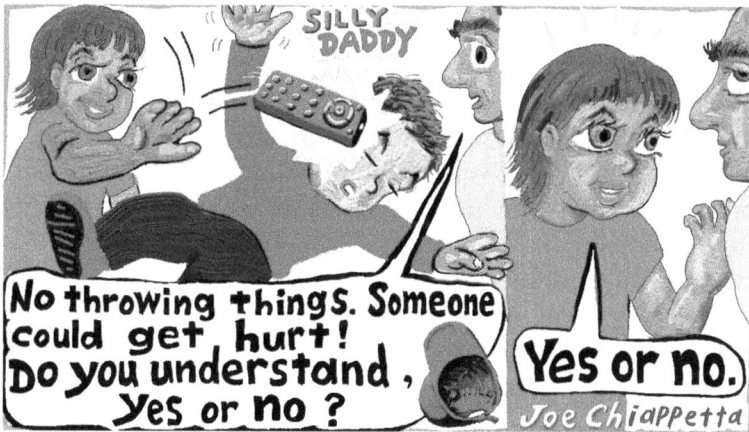

If you live long enough, it is likely you too will become disabled. Yet take heart--it is not likely that you'll ever be shot down by airplanes while climbing on top of a skyscraper. Sorry, King Kong.

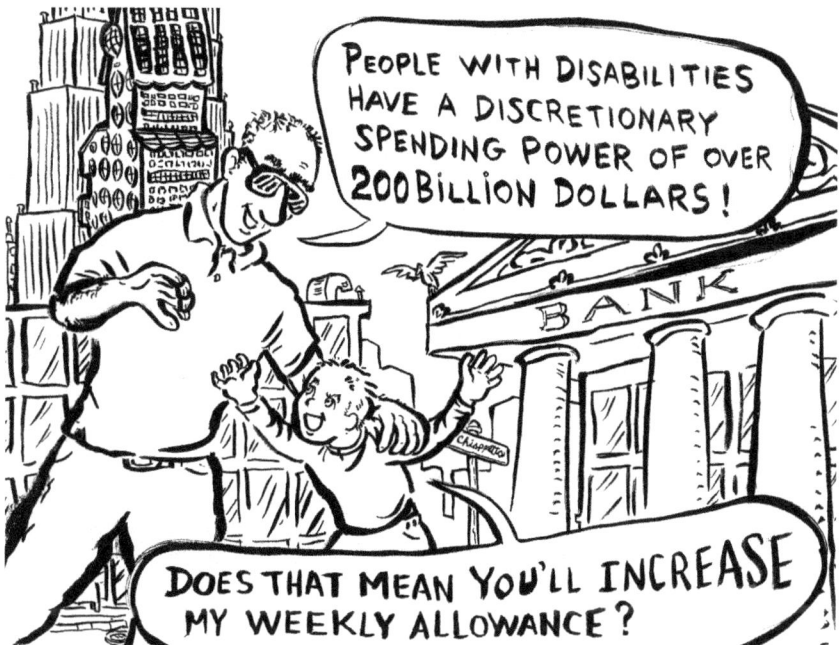

Despite living more than half of my entire life with a disability, it's remarkable how long I went without knowing anything about the disability population, or really anything about disability beyond my own pain and attempts at adaptation. When I first started working in the disability industry, I was overwhelmed with how many topics fall under the umbrella of disability. Some of these have already been mentioned, but there's a whole universe of disability "stuff" to digest. There are disability studies, disability statistics, disability funding, disability employment, disability advocacy, disability definitions, disability lawyers, disability etiquette, disability policy, disability community, and more. The list is seemingly endless as well as eye-opening.

I soon learned more about the connection between how work influences the growth of the mind, as well as inclusion into society. God designed us specifically to work, all the way on back to Adam and the beginnings of our history. Genesis 2:15 says **"The Lord God took the man and placed him in the garden of Eden to work it and watch over it."** Our creator designed us to work. Therefore, it naturally makes sense that work should be good for our continued mental health development.

In the book, *A History of Vocational Rehabilitation in America*, Doctor C. Esco Oberman touches on this subject as well.

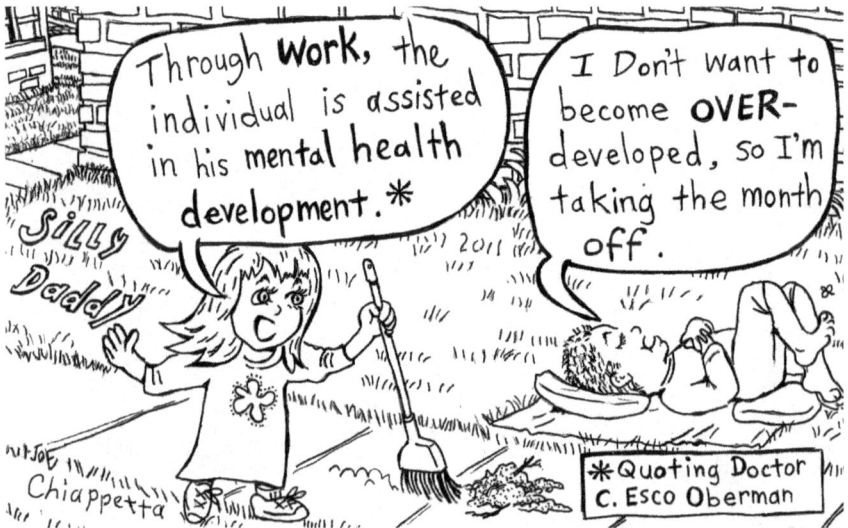

While the slacker gets his rest, the last laugh, of course, will be had by the people with jobs, money, and a disciplined lifestyle.

That's why it is essential that job seekers with disabilities be given equal opportunities for employment. Our mental health is at stake!

Think of how challenging it is to stay upbeat when you are unemployed and looking for a job. That's tough because so much of our sense of purpose is tied to what we do for a living and if we are appreciated. Our self image can really become scrambled when we can't connect with our purpose.

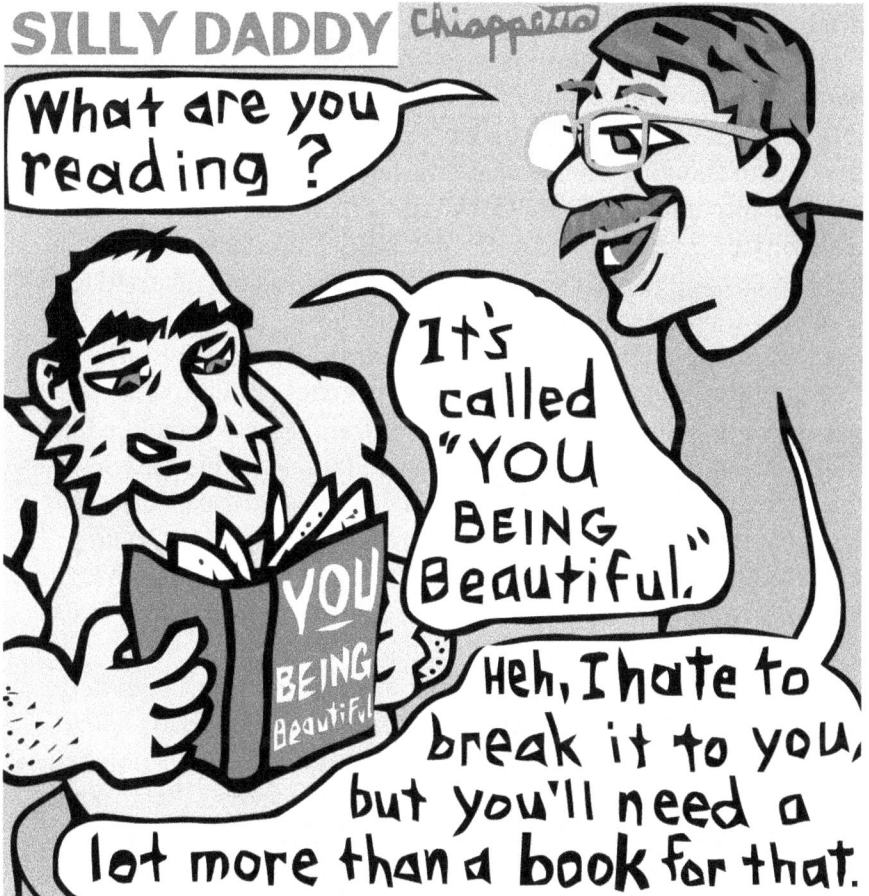

SILLY DADDY Chiappetta

What are you reading?

It's called "YOU BEING Beautiful."

YOU BEING Beautiful

Heh, I hate to break it to you, but you'll need a lot more than a book for that.

Moreover, as can be inferred from Dr. Oberman's writings on rehabilitation, if we don't work, we are in danger of becoming underdeveloped in the growth of our minds. Put simply, laziness is bad for you. So being unemployed is not a license to be lazy. That's the time to work even harder to find a job.

Once I began learning more deeply about employment topics as they relate to disability, I began to understand disability in a larger context. I started to appreciate the fact that I wasn't alone. Gradually, as I became fluent in more and more of the above-mentioned disability topics, I discovered that a whole new plane of existence opened up. Most people associate this borderless realm with the "disability rights movement." Certainly, that is a solid description, highlighting the fact that a select number of people with disabilities, their friends, and families, have loosely banded together to fight for fair treatment and equal prosperity for people with disabilities.

Nevertheless, I have a different name for this group of fighters. I affectionately refer to the realm where disability topics flow like fresh water from a mighty river as "Disability Geekdom." Like a band of computer geeks at a free high-tech hardware conference, Disability Geekdom is a place where every member is super-passionate about all things disability-related. The criteria for membership into Disability Geekdom is more than just having a disability or being a friend to the disability community. You also have to be excited to talk about disability issues, and unafraid to teach on it, whether formally or informally.

I still remember the day I entered Disability Geekdom. I was in the middle of conducting a disability awareness training for managers of about 10 retail stores. The training was scheduled later in the day, and it appeared as if the attendees were due for a nap. Therefore, to liven things up, I detached from my usual script and held my arms out wide, like a quarterback. "Look at me! Take a good look," I commanded. Then I slowly turned around without saying a word. Thereafter, I sat down and tested the crowd, "Raise your hand if you think I have a disability."

No matter what I said next, the training was instantly revitalized. Every attendee was fully alert now. Three people were even bold enough to raise their hand in answer to my question. The point was multidimensional. For the managers, they understood that disability is not about appearances, since many disabilities are non-apparent. It's about looking beyond the label and overcoming obstacles. For me, I understood that inspiring others about disability issues can be powerful and even has the potential to change the face of society. From that moment on, I became excited about conducting disability training and thus gained entrance into the halls of Disability Geekdom.

Despite the existence of Disability Geekdom, most people still have a fuzzy definition of what is and is not a disability. All too often, I've heard otherwise intelligent people assume things about disability that simply are not true. While listening to at least two speeches at disability events, I've raised an objectionable eyebrow when the speakers have said, "everyone has some sort of disability." Although I understand the importance of helping the general public understand that people with disabilities are just like everyone else, with highs and lows and in-betweens, the concept that everyone has a disability is simply not true.

There are only a few popularly accepted definitions of disability and none of them are aligned with the notion that all people have a disability. Let's look at the dominant definitions of disability.

The Americans with Disabilities Act of 1990 defined disability as the following:

"A physical or mental impairment that substantially limits one or more of the major life activities of such individual; a record of such an impairment; or being regarded as having such an impairment."

The U.S. Social Security Administration in 1956 defined disability in a different manner, tying it completely to the ability to make money:

"The law defines disability as the inability to engage in any substantial gainful activity by reason of any medically determinable physical or mental impairment(s) which can be expected to result in death or which has lasted or can be expected to last for a continuous period of not less than 12 months."

America certainly doesn't have the market cornered on disability terminology. The United Nations, through their World Health Organization, has a longer, yet very well thought-out definition of disability. Disability is **"an umbrella term for impairments, activity limitations and participation restrictions. Disability is the interaction between individuals with a health condition (e.g. cerebral palsy, Down syndrome and depression) and personal and environmental factors (e.g. negative attitudes, inaccessible transportation and public buildings, and limited social supports)."** I'm sure those in Disability Geekdom will want to look up their entire definition, assuming they haven't memorized it already. What I find most interesting about the definition coming out of the World Health Organization is that they also recognize in their 2011 *World Report on Disability* that disability is **"an evolving concept."**

While such knowledge salivates in minds throughout Disability Geekdom, a number of people unaware of this realm will try to assign disability status to conditions that usually are not actual disabilities. Once I had a conversation with a talented older woman who was having a hard time finding a job. She asked me if I could help, as she had been out of work for at least two years, looking for jobs the entire time. Since I have many contacts among agencies which assist people with disabilities in getting jobs, I asked her if she had a disability. If so, then I might be able to help.

Desperate for any assistance, she replied, "Well, isn't **age** a disability?"

"No," I answered, slightly surprised by her lack of awareness. Certainly the older you are, the more likely you are to acquire a disability. Yet in and of itself, age is not a disability.

Building upon a concept that cute people often appear more capable and less disabled, this imaginary encounter underscores some truths about human nature and disability. People with and without disabilities are widely uneducated about how to respond appropriately to disability issues. All too often, outward appearances largely influence how we think about other people. I have fallen into this deceptive trap too many times to count. Judging people's abilities based solely on how they look is not reliable and is potentially damaging.

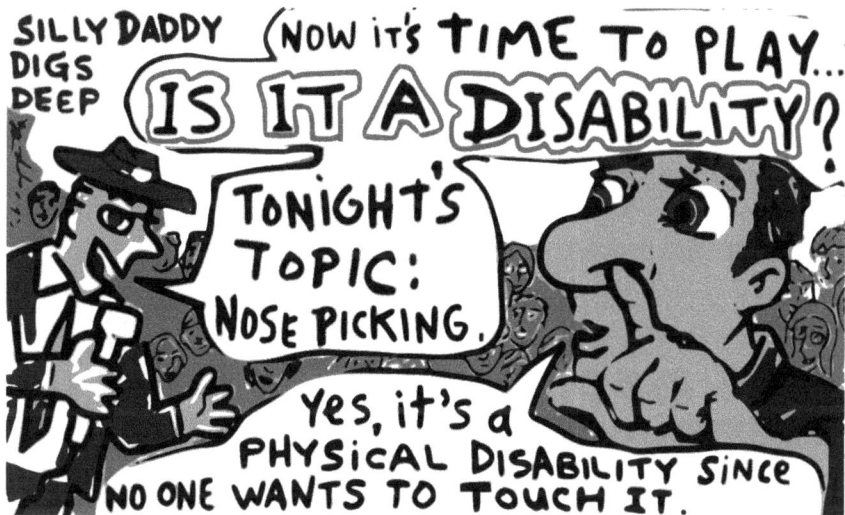

SILLY DADDY DIGS DEEP

NOW IT'S TIME TO PLAY...

IS IT A DISABILITY?

TONIGHT'S TOPIC: NOSE PICKING.

Yes, it's a PHYSICAL DISABILITY SINCE NO ONE WANTS TO TOUCH IT.

The multitude of misinterpretations regarding people's abilities and disability status has led me to occasionally maintain a silly mind game called "Is It a Disability?" The whole idea is to imagine an absurd human condition that comes into question as being a disability or not. Then ridiculous responses ensue. That's about the entire depth of the game. Despite the absurdity of this activity, it helps me to remember not to get caught up in labels and outward appearances.

I'm so grateful for the few people who did not cave in to judging me by my looks when I was in the worst episodes of back pain. Most people would be less likely to regard me as fully capable while I frequently had a grimace of pain on my face. Yet even in the depths of my disability, I was still called to useful and even noble purposes.

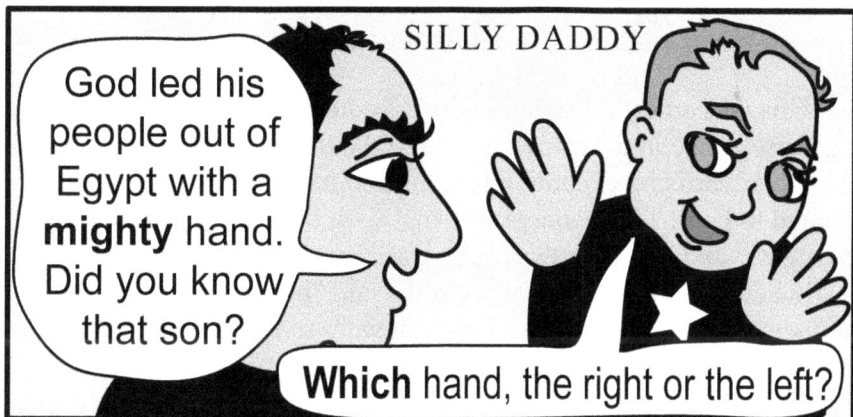

SILLY DADDY

God led his people out of Egypt with a **mighty** hand. Did you know that son?

Which hand, the right or the left?

Being a good parent, managing the Chicago International Christian Church website, training companies on disability awareness, and being faithful to God remained core duties in my life. Through it all, I've learned that disability is about embracing responsibility despite the obstacles. The journey has tested and refined me, along with countless other folks, I imagine. So bring on another day in Disability Geekdom.

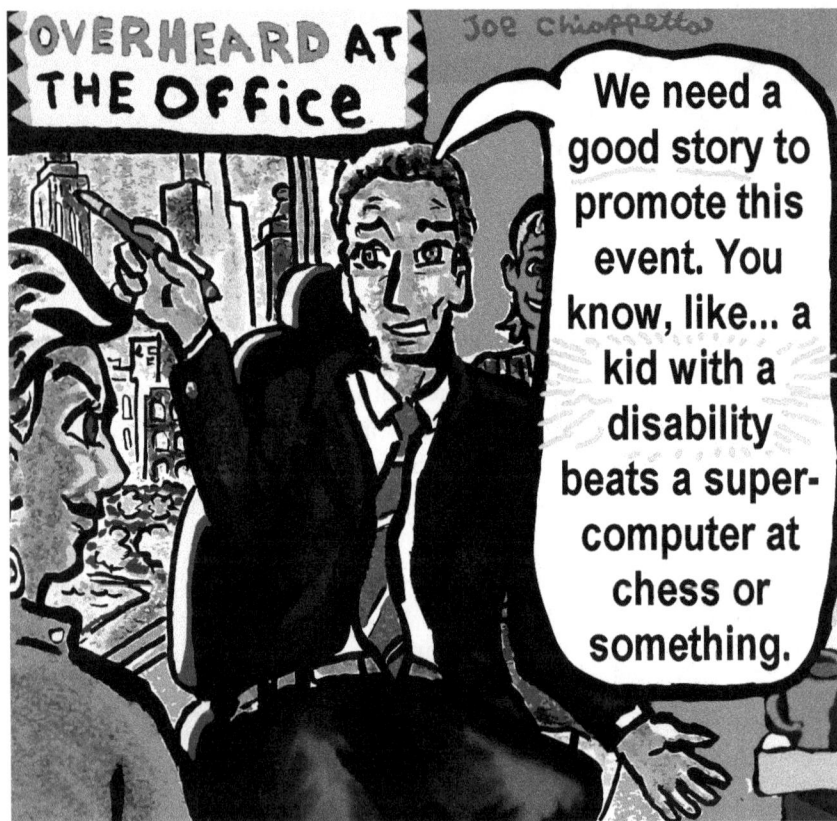

This was an actual statement that I couldn't help but overhear at a high-rise office in downtown Chicago. With the confidence of a rock star, an advertising executive told his clients exactly what they wanted to hear. This concept was met with favorable feedback like, "Alright!" and "Yeah, let's do it!"

In actuality, the ad executive truly said "handicapped kid" in his moment of "inspiration," but I did not want to further popularize that label. The term "handicapped" is now seen by most people with disabilities as a derogatory term, as in "poor beggar with your *cap* in your *hand*."

Here is a bonus quiz for those wanting to test their knowledge. There is a profound moral to this supercomputer comic. Please choose the moral of the story. Select your best answer from a list of multiple choices:

A) Kids with disabilities are smarter than you.

B) Don't let advertising executives have a strong influence over the world, or anything really.

C) If you had a supercomputer, you wouldn't waste time playing chess with it. Bring on the multi-player online 3D shooting games.

D) A better story would involve pirates, robots, and ninjas with disabilities.

E) Business people know what they are talking about and wearing a suit validates everything they say.

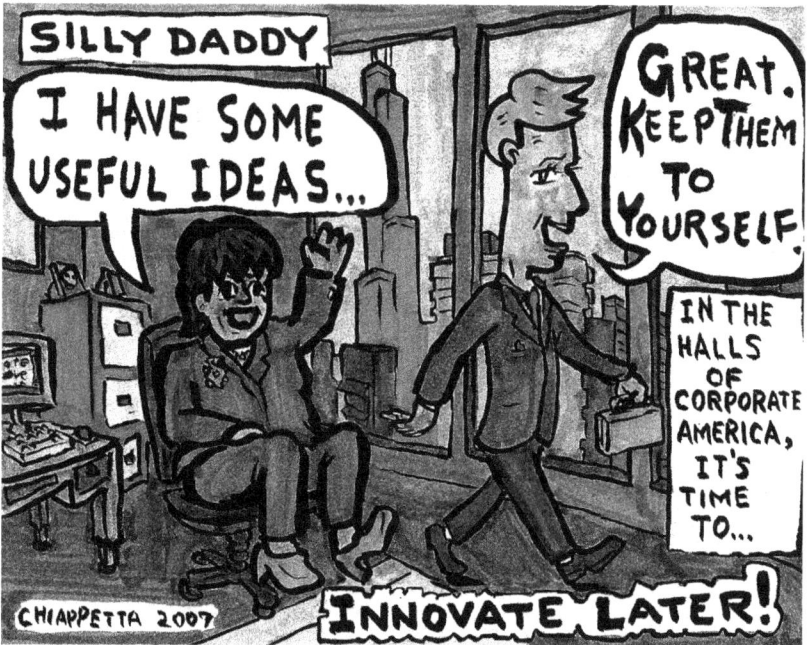

Chapter 8:

The System Is Not Your Friend

After sitting through many long speeches by disability experts salted with accolades to each other, when pressed for real solutions to societal problems, little has been widely effective regarding disability employment. Through the years, I have all too often gotten the sense that many paid experts and consultants tell you three types of information:

    1) Information that you already know.

    2) Information that you could frequently figure out without them.

    3) Information that someone else has already been paid to discover and make public.

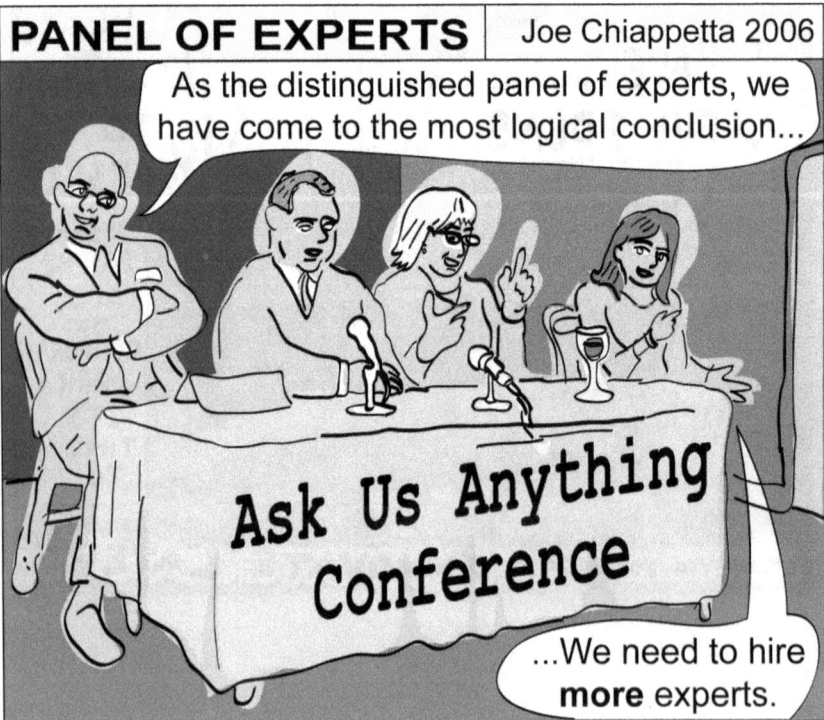

I bring this up partly because **"there is nothing new under the sun,"** as stated throughout Ecclesiastes. I also bring this up because I believe the disability-employment field is suffering from what's known as the "paralysis of analysis." I wish I could say this is shocking, but many high-powered disability leaders are too reliant on expensive surveys that tell us what is already known, yet change nothing. Recently, one group even had the nerve to fund disability-employment research about other disability research! To add insult to injury, the disability community is praising this as important and newsworthy. I, however, see it as intellectuals getting drunk on their own fruit punch. It's too bad we couldn't take all the money poured into disability-employment research over the last two decades and just give it to people with disabilities to start their own businesses.

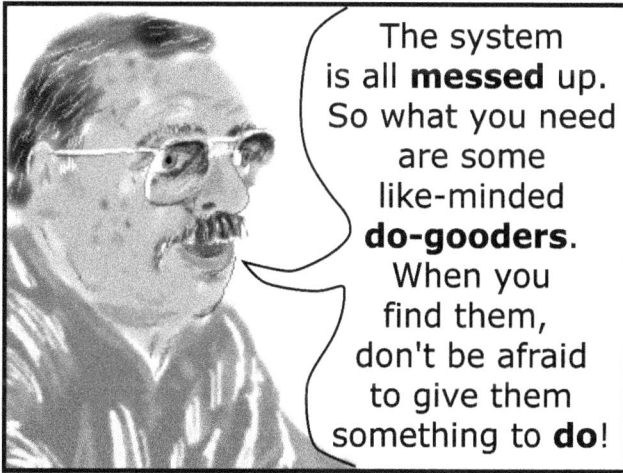

The system is all **messed** up. So what you need are some like-minded **do-gooders**. When you find them, don't be afraid to give them something to **do**!

Put simply, there is too much talk and not enough action. An old mentor in the disability-employment arena once told me something very useful. Speaking on community organizing around disability-employment, he knew how to cut right to the chase.

Many of his statements were very wise, and more leaders would do well to call the like-minded do-gooders to action. Part of my attempt at helping people with disabilities involves leading and managing a network of workforce developers who, in turn, help people with disabilities find jobs. I have been in this role for about a decade, and over one thousand people with disabilities have found jobs through the collaborations maintained in this group.

Due to this success, my position and this network have received a decent amount of attention from various local governments, and I frequently find myself pulled onto one disability-employment committee or another. Recently, I was on a big conference call about how the government is supposed to be helping people with disabilities find jobs. Disability policy leaders were verbally glad-handing each other over the phone about how great they are and what a pleasure it is to be working together. It was so hard to stomach. Employment support systems for people with disabilities are messed up beyond repair. The entire system needs to be trashed and rebuilt from the ground up.

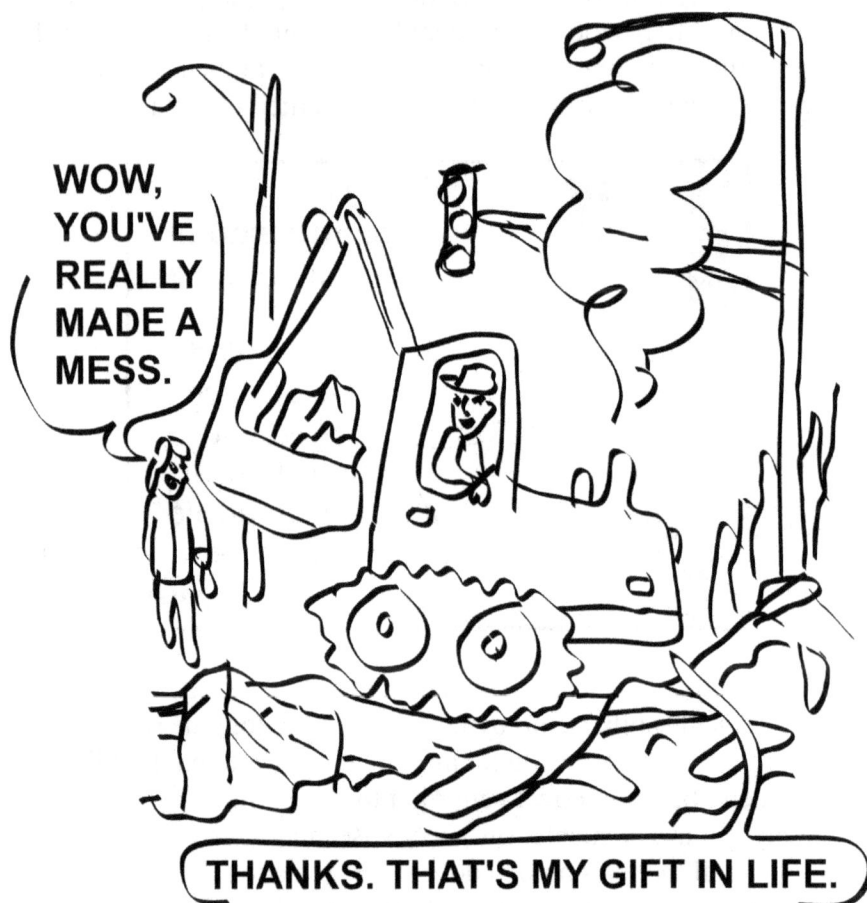

WOW, YOU'VE REALLY MADE A MESS.

THANKS. THAT'S MY GIFT IN LIFE.

Destroying the current system is counted as fighting words for the entrenched bureaucrats who don't want to rock the boat. Yet it is the truth. The proof is in the fact that the unemployment rate of people with disabilities has not improved significantly in any of the decades since the passing of the Americans with Disabilities Act of 1990. Fewer jobs for people with disabilities means more poverty for them. With great directness, Chicago's commissioner of the Mayor's Office for People with Disabilities has spoken publicly about the link between disability and poverty.

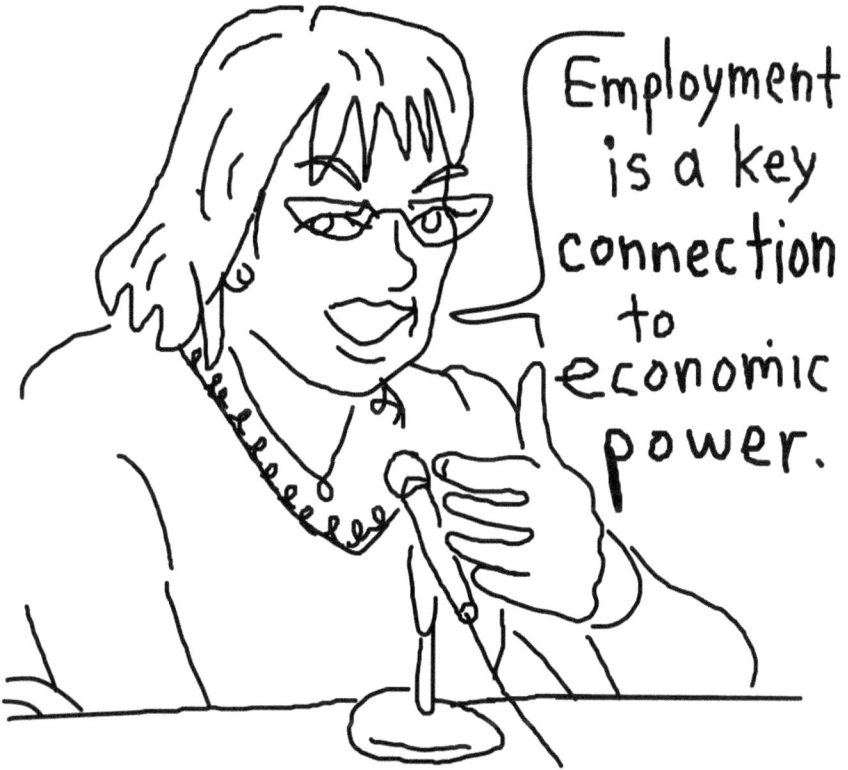

Employment is a key connection to economic power.

Outside of my workforce developer network, which has modest, yet consistent local success placing people with disabilities in jobs, what else should be done to improve employment options for people with disabilities? I have prayed for clarity on this complex issue. My gut keeps telling me that everything--and I do mean everything-- needs to change. Business, government, education, and nonprofits are all part of the problem, with no viable and comprehensive solution in sight.

Despite the endless amount of hype generated by organizations to secure more deals and funding, most groups are internally aware of their inability to create lasting change. In fact, when most of these organizations speak off the record, they freely admit that they are only scratching the surface and many are struggling to keep their doors open.

Doing more with less is what most of these organizations are forced into due to funding cuts. The problem with doing more with less is that it only works when you have great workers with better ideas. Sadly, this is rarely the case in organizations. What is more likely to happen is the creation of top heavy organizations with low-paid frontline workers doing more with not just less, but with little experience or real world clout. That's a recipe for disaster. Without a brilliant plan and brilliant workers, more with less gives way to burnt out workers and sub-par services. Everybody loses.

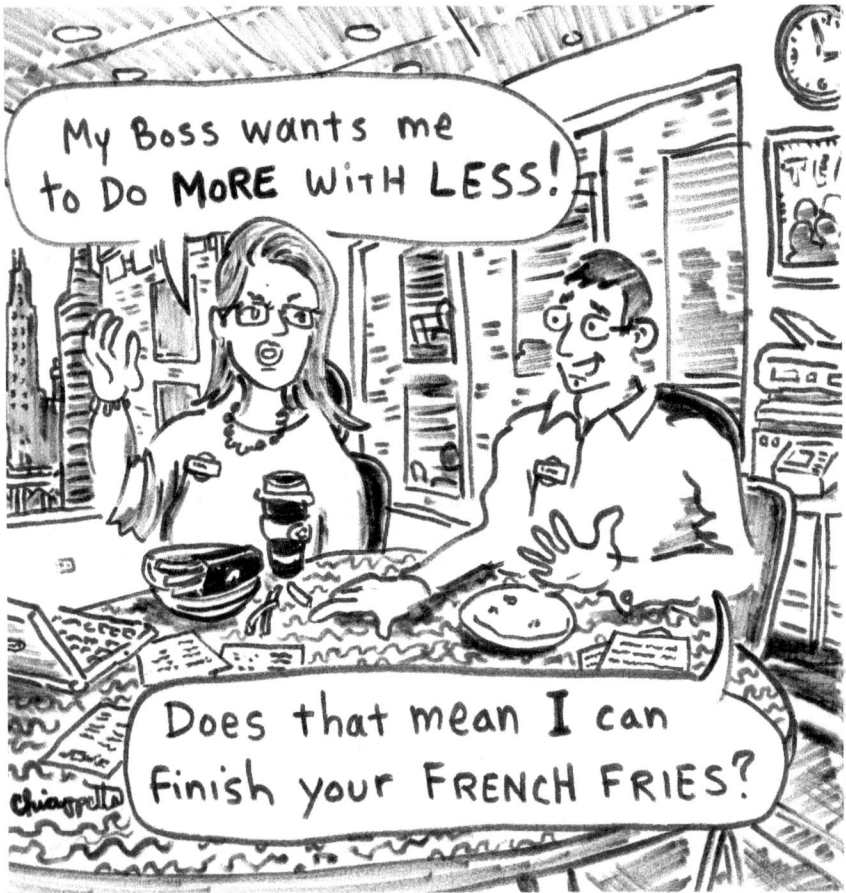

Helping one person at a time, some of these groups are able to have a minor local impact, and I know they have a number of grateful customers. Nevertheless, they're all operating in a toxic employment-placement arena that will never solve systemic problems. It's like doctors who just treat symptoms, yet never offer the cure. That has got to change.

Consider this parallel: people with chronic pain need healing rather than mere temporary relief. In much the same way, job seekers with disabilities don't merely need help finding one job. Rather, they need a national employment culture that will fully embrace and even seek them out as employees.

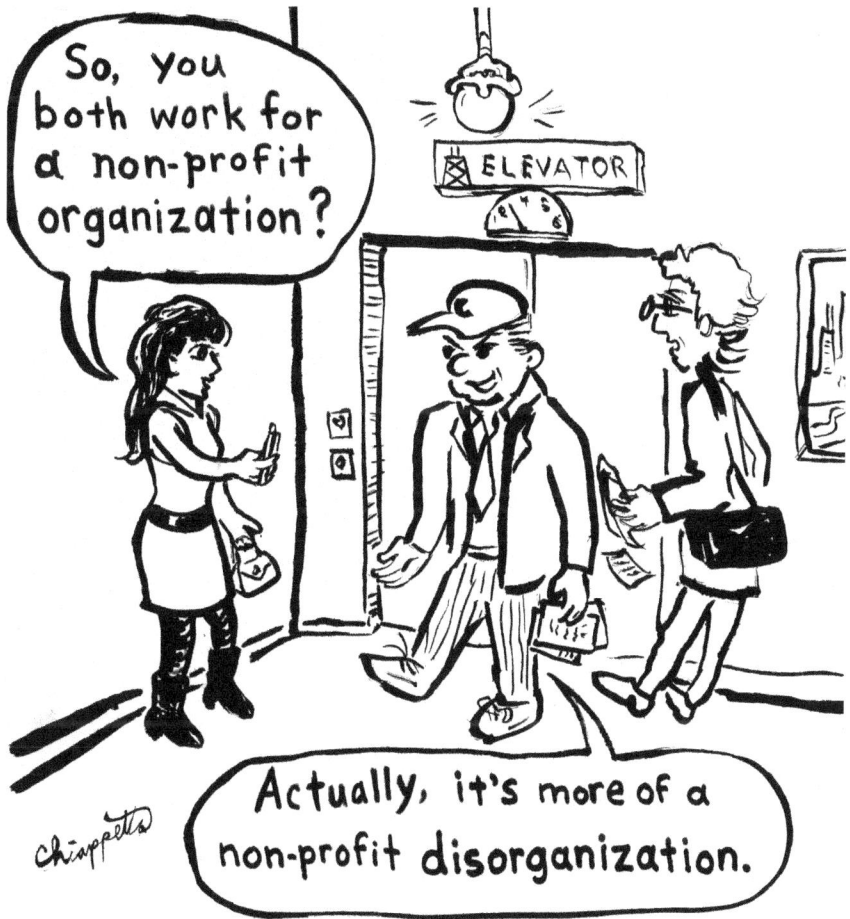

Due to this proliferation of visionless bureaucracies and groups operating mainly as another mouth to feed, and thus being part of the problem, I am offering a solution that I believe will be the most direct way to fix the issue of low employment for people with disabilities. The solution is as simple as it is radical. It involves three bold steps intentionally designed to destroy the current ineffective disability-employment industry and create a new process that cuts out the middlemen and pays companies directly for results. I call this plan "**Disability Employment Cash for Companies**."

1) Amend the laws to make the following activities legal.

2) Withdraw all money that goes to fund government and non-profit job placement programs that help people with disabilities find jobs. In the USA, that's currently over 3 billion dollars for vocational rehabilitation and research.

3) Use all of that money to directly pay employers to hire people with disabilities. Specifically, this would be upfront payment, not tax breaks, to companies who hire workers with disabilities as well as upfront payment to companies who retain workers with disabilities for one year. With 3 billion dollars annually available, 750,000 workers with disabilities per year could come with $4,000 in hiring incentives each.

Right about now, most non-profit professionals with rehabilitation counseling expertise should be crying, "What about our jobs?" Good question. The job placement side of the rehabilitation industry should be completely dismantled. People with disabilities aren't hungry for counseling. They're hungry for employers who offer them jobs. Therefore, only the hard-working all-stars in the rehabilitation placement field should continue their work, but not for government or non-profits. Rather, they should go to work for the employers to help them maximize their recruitment of people with disabilities from inside the company.

For too long I have observed too many rehabilitation professionals with little business sense fumble with for-profit companies because they're too comfortable in counselor mode. Approaching businesses scares them or they're just burnt out. Many in vocational rehabilitation think they deserve to be pushing pencils in a quiet office while admiring their fancy degree and telling job seekers with disabilities things they've heard a thousand times. Therefore, with a "Disability Employment Cash for Companies" plan, those days of waste would be over.

While in-depth details of this plan are not the topic of this book, I am certain such a plan would stimulate the economy and create attractive reasons to hire and retain workers with disabilities. Employment cultures would shift to environments wherein recruitment and competition to find, employ, and train workers with disabilities would be aggressive, solution-oriented, and business-driven. These are the very features that disability-employment industry insiders have talked about for decades, yet consistently fail to deliver on, year after year.

I have discussed this plan with a few disability-employment leaders already, yet so far, the response has been met with odd curiosity and the following attitudes:

"It certainly would shake things up, and it might work, but the entire government would have to change to support such an effort."

"You need more research to prove your case. Otherwise, it will be impossible to get people on board."

"You realize that you'd be shooting yourself, and the entire vocational rehabilitation industry in the foot, don't you?"

"That plan is way beyond our scope of work."

"Well, you could write a grant and see if some foundation would fund a small demonstration version of this."

The most interesting thing about these comments is that no one said it couldn't work. Moreover, I have faith that my proposal will eventually be implemented and hiring managers will one day accept and embrace results-driven business payments to hire people with disabilities--even people with severe disabilities. If there is money involved, my experience has been that business people will find ways to make it work.

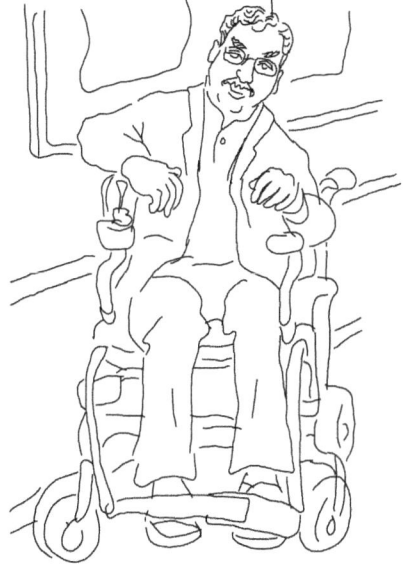

Nevertheless, even if no one adopts my proposal, I am sure that Jesus can fix the unemployment problem for people with disabilities. The real question is this: who is turning to him? I, for one, will continue to pray and promote better employment opportunities for people with disabilities. I do wonder what God thinks of all the untapped potential of people with disabilities? They (we) are all too frequently marginalized by society. Someday in heaven, disability will not matter. Until then, I imagine that it will be a hard fight and a hard, yet gratifying life for those who seek and find God, as well as a decent job.

Reflecting upon disability from a spiritual perspective, an ironic concept occurs to me. Jesus, the savior and lamb of God, did his most impressive and hope-giving acts while nailed to a cross! If that is not a disability, then I don't know what is. Such a thought gives me comfort. God's plan of redemption was only made possible by Jesus while he had acquired multiple disabilities as the crucified son of God. A careful reading of Jesus' last day before he died reveals that he endured bloody sweat, also known as hematidrosis, a Roman flogging, punches, a crown of thorns, and pierced hands and feet.

Therefore, it was with multiple disabilities that Jesus took upon himself the sins of the world.

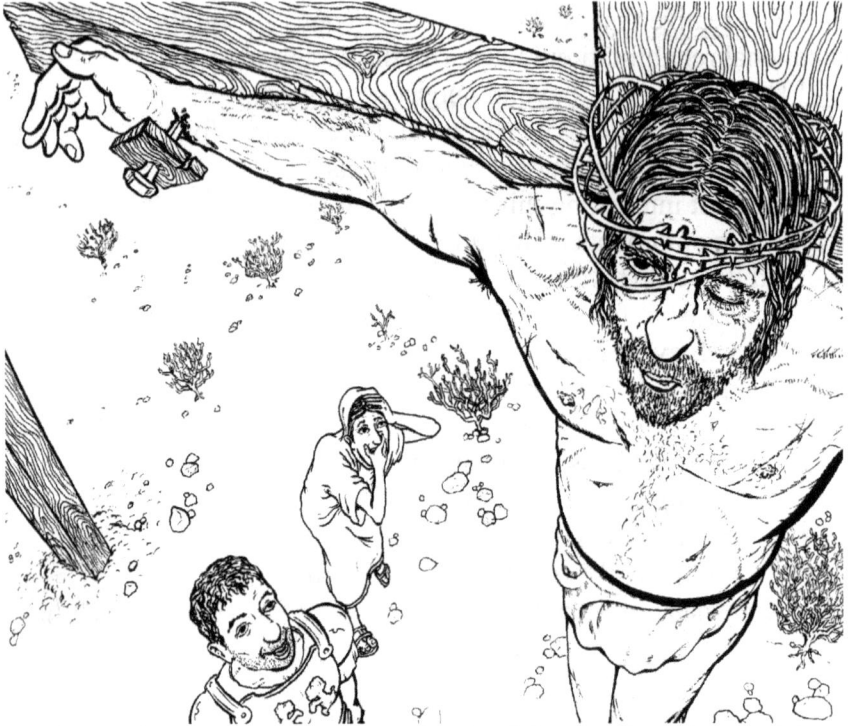

Then, of course, he rose from the dead. Being dead is certainly another disability, to say the least. However, Jesus did not let the tragedy of his death stop him from overcoming the impossible. The resurrection is proof that messed-up situations can change.

The challenge for me is to choose to be hopeful and solution-oriented about the discrimination against people with disabilities. A resurrection mindset must prevail despite all the barriers set up in our aging and imperfect bodies, which are really only a temporary dwelling for our souls. If Jesus conquered death, then surely with his guidance, we can resurrect the dismal employment outlook for the millions of people with disabilities out there who may or may not have the mercy to look upon unfair hiring practices and say to employers, **"Father, forgive them, for they know not what they do."** (Luke 23:34)

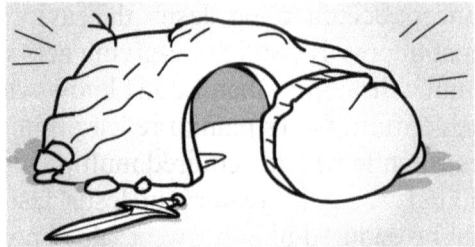

Chapter 9:

A Funny Thing Happened while Exercising

Throughout the years living with a back injury, I have always been told by countless medical professionals, as well as armchair advisors, to exercise. This was after I told them the usual: that it is painful for me to sit for more than five minutes at a time, that sometimes I can hardly even walk, and that lifting is painful. After countless examinations, the paid experts told me I had arthritis, a herniated disc, degenerative disc disease, a neurological disorder, or weak stomach muscles. So I have gone through all sorts of varied workouts prescribed therein.

These workouts, while useful for physical activity, never actually healed me. They strengthened me, and gave me time to think, but I still had the same issues with not being able to sit without pain. However, I have found it most ironic that often what is said while I am working out can bring both comic relief as well as chronic relief. It's hard to be in pain when you're laughing, and soon I realized that state of mind has everything to do with healing.

One such funny comment occurred while I was doing sit-ups. This was during my regular morning exercises, when my two-year-old daughter joined in on the fun, which is amusing in and of itself, if you've ever seen a toddler try to do a workout.

She didn't say so directly, but

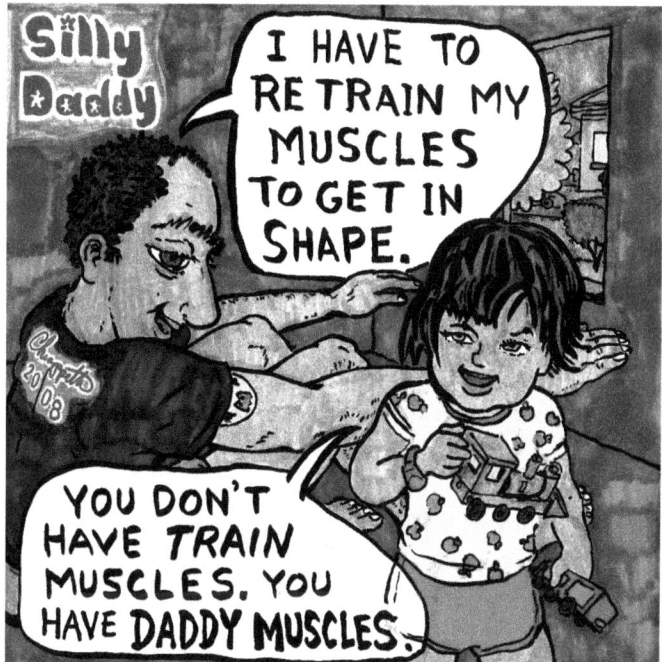

in her eyes, I was not disabled--I was strong. I was her daddy.

73

Having someone believe in you is an important part of the rehabilitation process. My daughter believed in me and made me laugh as well.

Another time, in the middle of some stretching exercises using a giant plastic workout ball, I was talking with my little daughter and saw the resemblance of my wife in my baby's face. There's something about working out with family that calls forth the extra intensity of life.

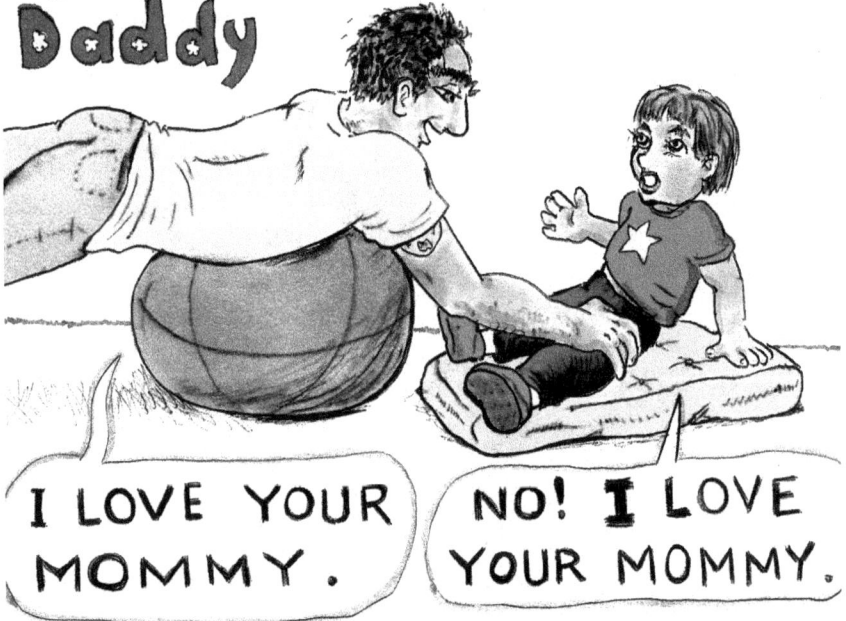

Using humor to deal with serious health issues seems to be a tactic that a good number of people with disabilities put into practice. Visiting her grandfather in the hospital recently, after he almost died, my youngest daughter presented him with something she had made to encourage him. Her grandfather certainly liked the drawing, since what grandparent doesn't treasure the little things that their little ones make for them as gifts? Ironically though, her grandfather was all the more enthusiastic to make jokes about his situation rather than face the grim seriousness of the events that led him to his dire health condition.

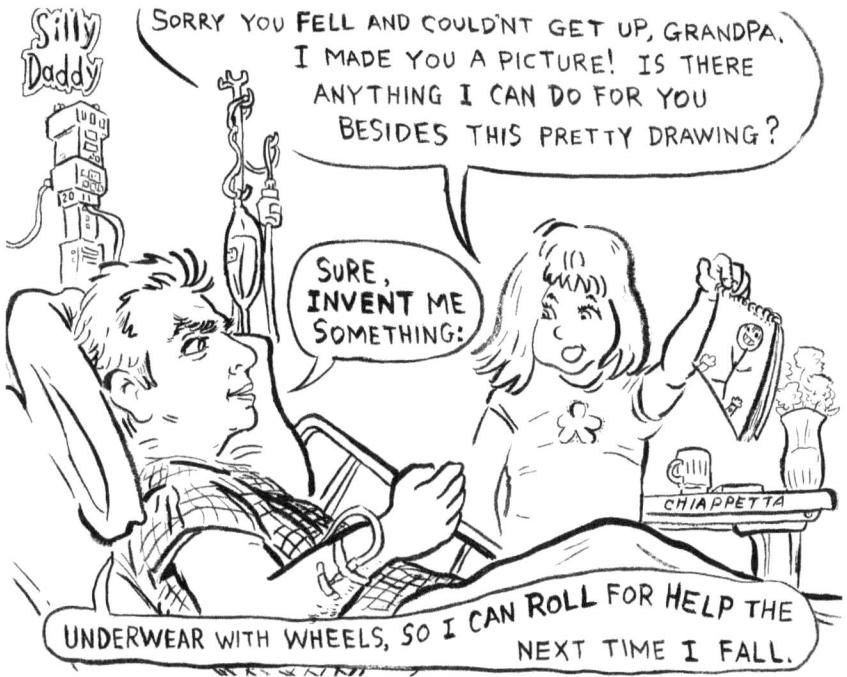

Working out with my son, all sorts of amusing comments also get invented. The following discussion took place when he was five years old.

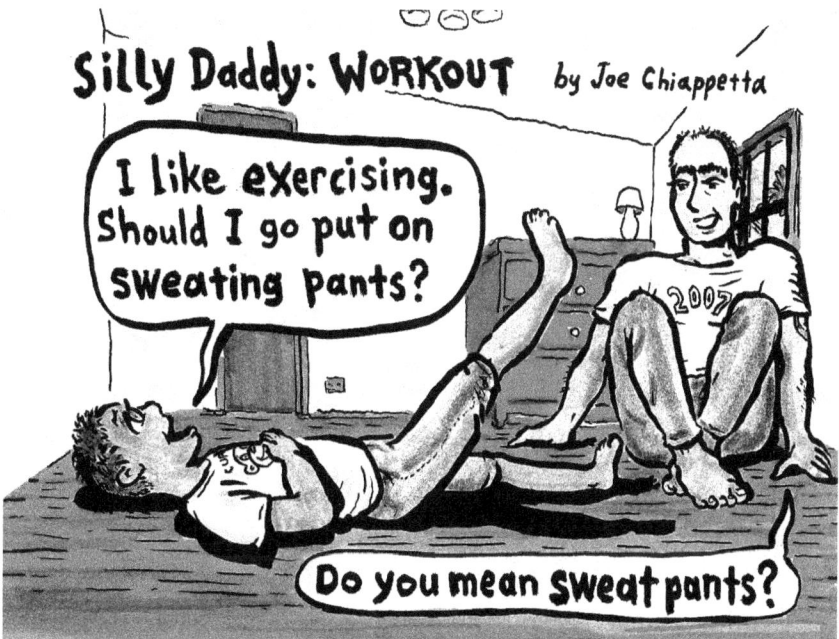

This comical scene became a household influence in no time. Now the whole family calls sweatpants by its more action-oriented name: "sweating pants," just for fun. If only I could wear sweating pants to the office. They're so much more comfortable.

On a different occasion, while doing push-ups with my son when he was seven, another timeless talk took place.

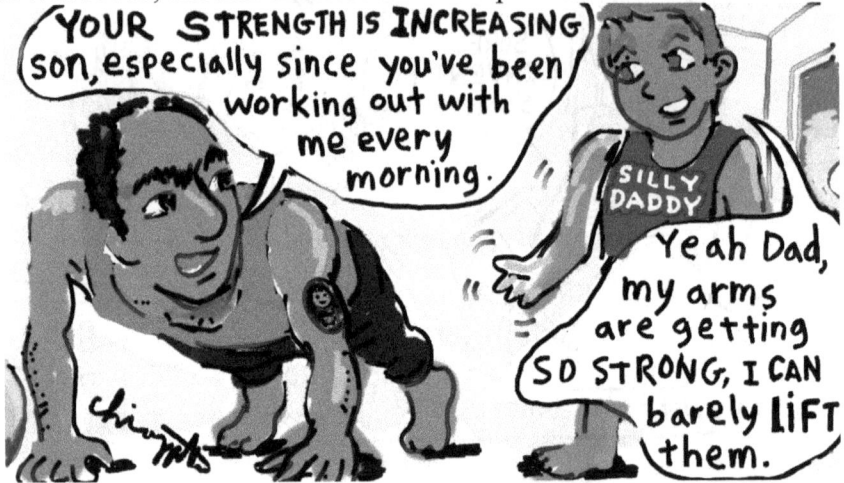

YOUR STRENGTH IS INCREASING son, especially since you've been working out with me every morning.

SILLY DADDY

Yeah Dad, my arms are getting SO STRONG, I CAN barely LIFT them.

Waking up extra early to pray, read the Bible, and then exercise takes mental discipline that can be hard to maintain over long periods of time. I found that if I occupied my mind with prayer, as well as humor, the tough workouts passed a lot quicker.

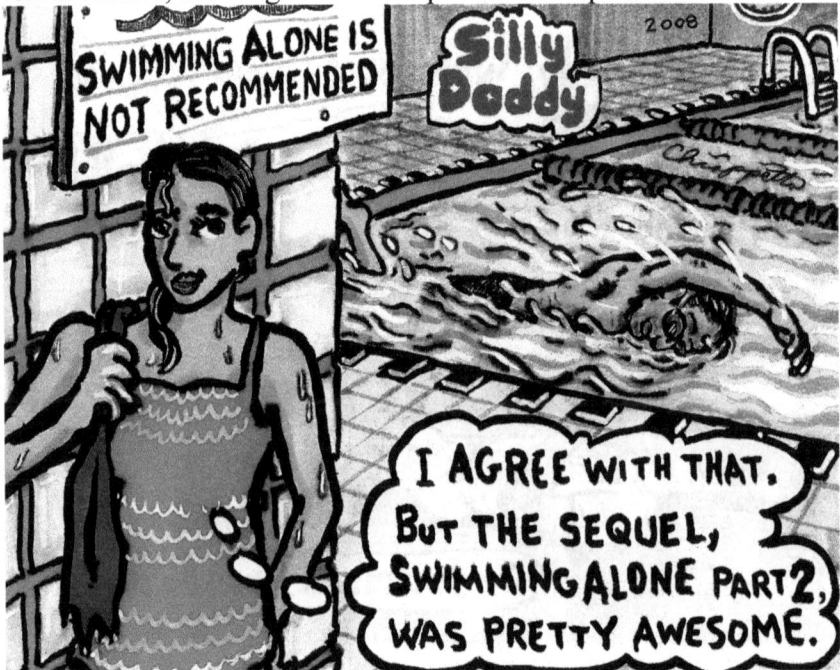

SWIMMING ALONE IS NOT RECOMMENDED

Silly Daddy

2008

I AGREE WITH THAT. BUT THE SEQUEL, SWIMMING ALONE PART 2, WAS PRETTY AWESOME.

On one such occasion, while swimming to strengthen my muscles, I kept getting distracted by the warning sign in the pool room. It read "Swimming Alone Is Not Recommended." Therefore, I imagined the health club management making all sorts of recommendations, and perhaps they'd be posting book reviews too.

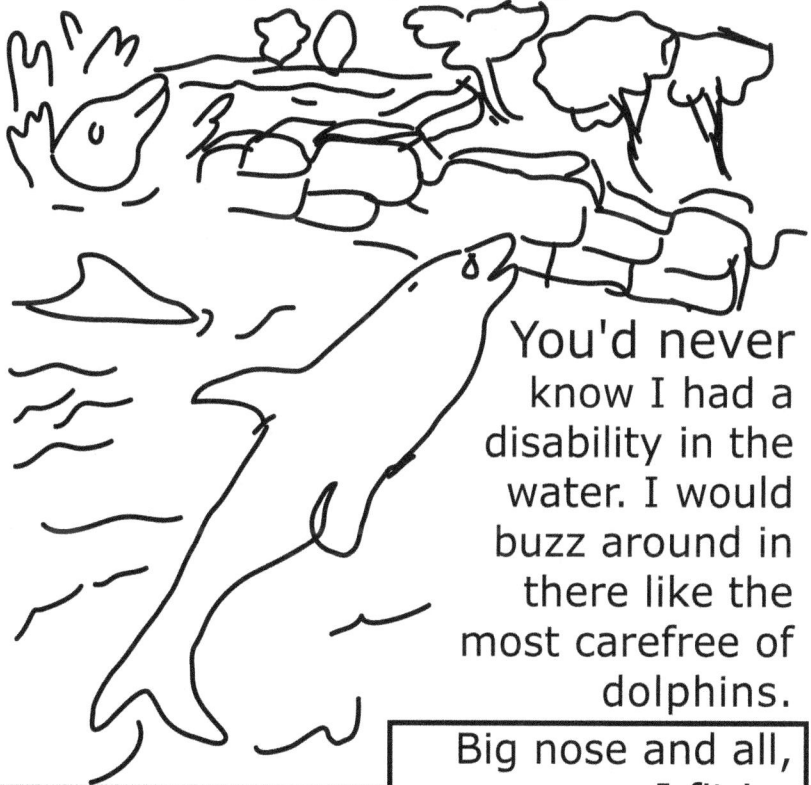

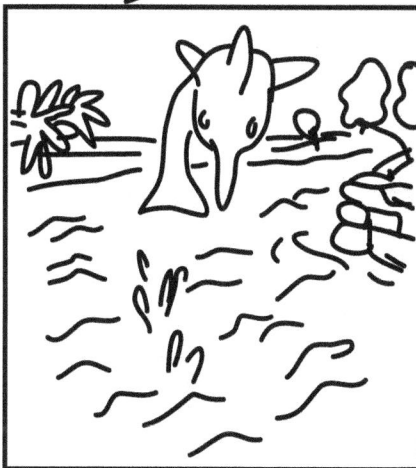

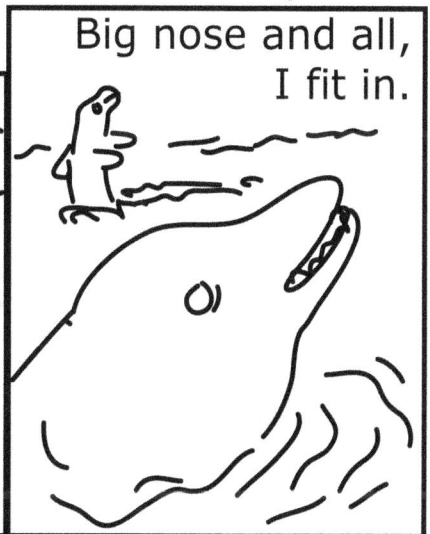

You'd never know I had a disability in the water. I would buzz around in there like the most carefree of dolphins.

Big nose and all, I fit in.

All this and more was dreamed up during my weekly training sessions at the Lakeshore Athletic Club swimming pool in Chicago.

At the time, I was doing ten laps about three days a week. Those workouts produced in me a renewed belief that I could still engage in rigorous physical activity. At least there was some place on the earth that I could float on equal footing with others--in the water.

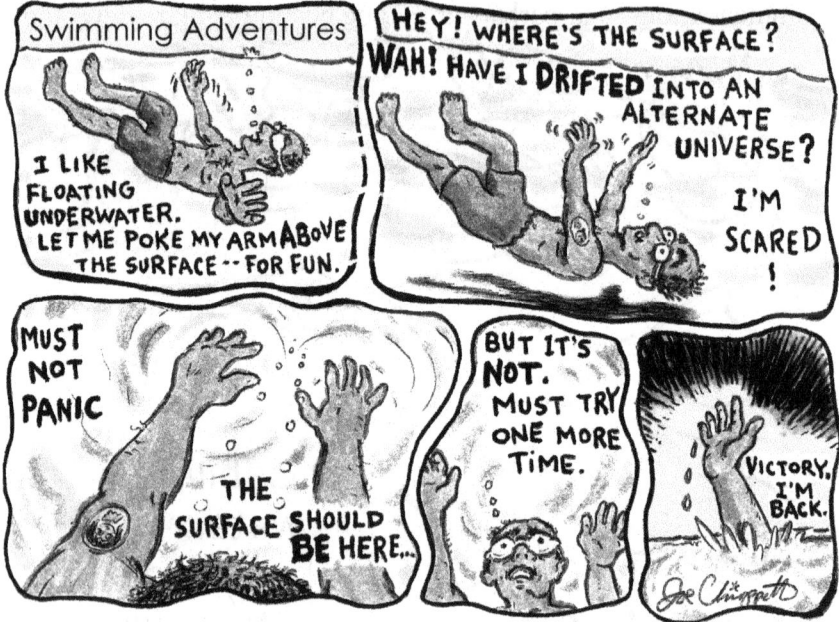

My pool workouts produced all sorts of creative concepts. Something about being in water and doing laps over and over shifted my thinking in a unique way--making it literally more fluid.

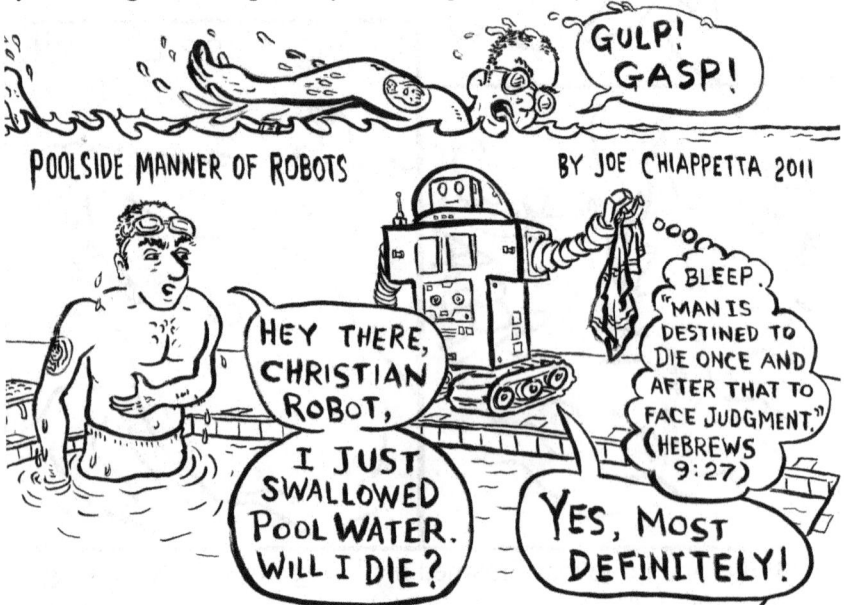

I think it was in the pool that I came up with a comic character named "Christian Robot." On one such occasion, I accidentally gulped a lot of water while doing the freestyle swimming stroke. This was toward the end of my workout routine, and I was also feeling the irritation of the pool's chlorine in my system. So I would ask questions that were really on my mind to my trusted Bible-processing imaginary robot friend. The combination of physical activity with spiritually-engaging meditation--silly as some of mine appeared to be--was often highly invigorating.

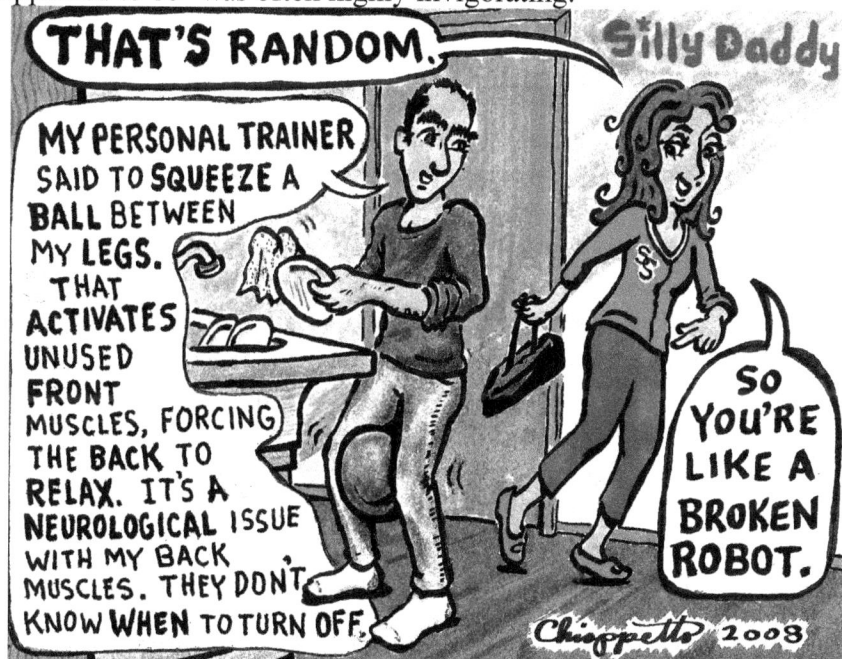

THAT'S RANDOM, Silly Daddy

MY PERSONAL TRAINER SAID TO SQUEEZE A BALL BETWEEN MY LEGS. THAT ACTIVATES UNUSED FRONT MUSCLES, FORCING THE BACK TO RELAX. IT'S A NEUROLOGICAL ISSUE WITH MY BACK MUSCLES. THEY DON'T KNOW WHEN TO TURN OFF.

SO YOU'RE LIKE A BROKEN ROBOT.

Chiappette 2008

Also exercise-related, my wife and I have a friend from church named Lisa Fellis, who unknowingly prompted me to eventually see something quite helpful about the nature of disability issues. I will explain this in more detail later, because the helpful nature of her statement didn't occur to me when she first called me a "broken robot." Due to the rapid fire of her witty comments, we sometimes refer to Lisa as "Silly Sister." It's a name she certainly has earned.

Regarding this particular exercise, squeezing a ball really hard, as it was placed between my knees, actually made the back pain temporarily go away. It was baffling, but true. The problem, however, was that I couldn't very well squeeze a ball between my legs all day.

Yet I learned so much from the personal trainer who showed me that exercise. Justin was his name. Everything he told me was confirmed in things I would come to understand only later. He said I should not think like I am stuck with the same weak muscles and bad joints for the rest of my life. That simply was not true. The body, he explained, was constantly in a state of regeneration--that is how it is designed. What we put into the body and how we use the body makes all the difference in how the body heals. Justin's workout plan, while it did not bring complete healing, brought me from a dismal 25 percent functionality up to about 75 percent functionality. Before I started working with Justin, I could not sit for more than a few minutes without pain. Yet after a few weeks on Justin's workout, I could sit pain-free for 45 minutes, and even drive for an hour with only minor discomfort. That's progress.

The reason why special thanks also go to Lisa, also known as Silly Sister, for actually having the nerve to call me a "broken robot" to my face, is a bit complex. The statement, aside from being hilarious, helped me to grasp how other people might see me. The fact that Lisa was able to acknowledge my disability in a light-hearted way, without making a big deal about it, was important. For the first time thereafter, I realized that if she could accept my disability and move on, then perhaps others could too--not just with regard to me, but for all people with disabilities.

For the record, I'm not suggesting that people with disabilities should now be regarded as broken robots. Yet for me, something clicked here. Lisa knew that I think robots are pretty cool, broken or otherwise. What she said taught me there were things I could do or communicate to make disability issues more acceptable and engaging for people without disabilities. I call this my "broken robot" moment. Taking the fear out of disability issues and replacing it with light-hearted understanding will go a long way to helping employers embrace more people with disabilities in the workplace.

It should come as no surprise that shortly after the broken robot moment, I started speaking publicly about my own disability to companies in efforts to make employers more "disability aware." Executives and managers from Walgreens, Manpower, and many other companies heard directly from me on how to be amused and enthused about hiring people with disabilities. These talks led to direct hires of people with disabilities into these huge corporations. Not bad for a broken robot.

Despite many challenges and life adjustments, my wife Denise was incredibly supportive throughout this whole process. She also amazed me for her ability to keep a sharp sense of humor about the whole disability issue.

Early on, after one of the first times that I came home from my athletic club workout, with a sense of accomplishment, I told my wife about my workout, and she surprised me with one of her classic unorthodox comments.

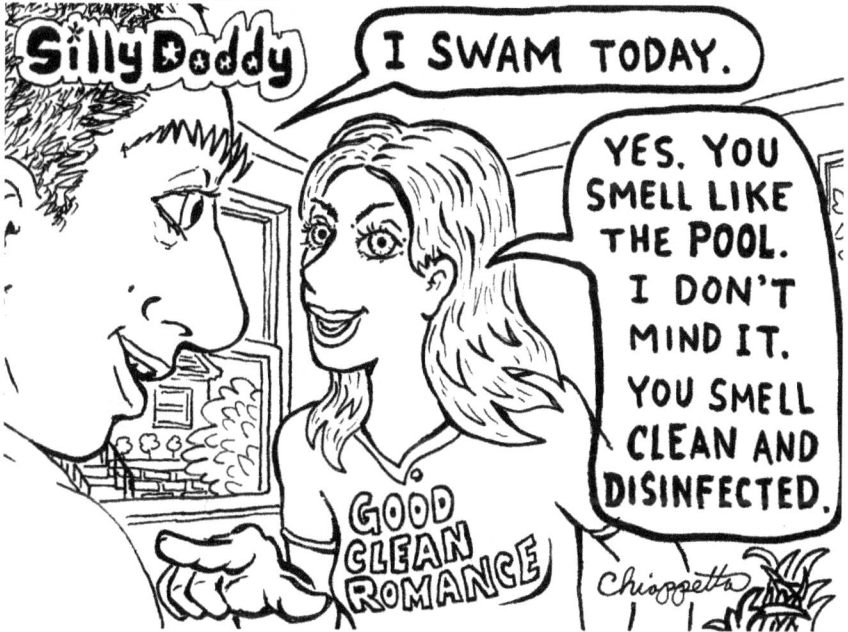

With both humor and encouragement, my wife and other close friends never gave up on me. This was a beacon of light for my soul. The key in all those situations was seeing and helping others to see the abilities in people, not the impairments. Retrain your mind to look for what a person can do--not what they can't do--in any situation.

There are examples of this all over in everyday life. Once, on a downtown Chicago city train platform, I crouched down to take a closer look at a pinkish-gray little creature and realized that the featured animal was different from his fellows. It was a bird limping not unlike Charlie Chaplin, the old actor from black and white films. The bird's feet were stumps--like a mini rhino. The poor guy had no claws. I couldn't even imagine what had happened to make the bird this way. Had he been born that way, or was it a disease, or worse; did some foe bite them off in a life-and-death conflict? Whatever the case, the poor bird could not walk like everyone else. I quickly wondered what other functional limitations the bird might be stuck with. Perhaps his wings don't work as well. It's a miracle he's survived this long in the big city. Surely, though, this fellow's days must be numbered.

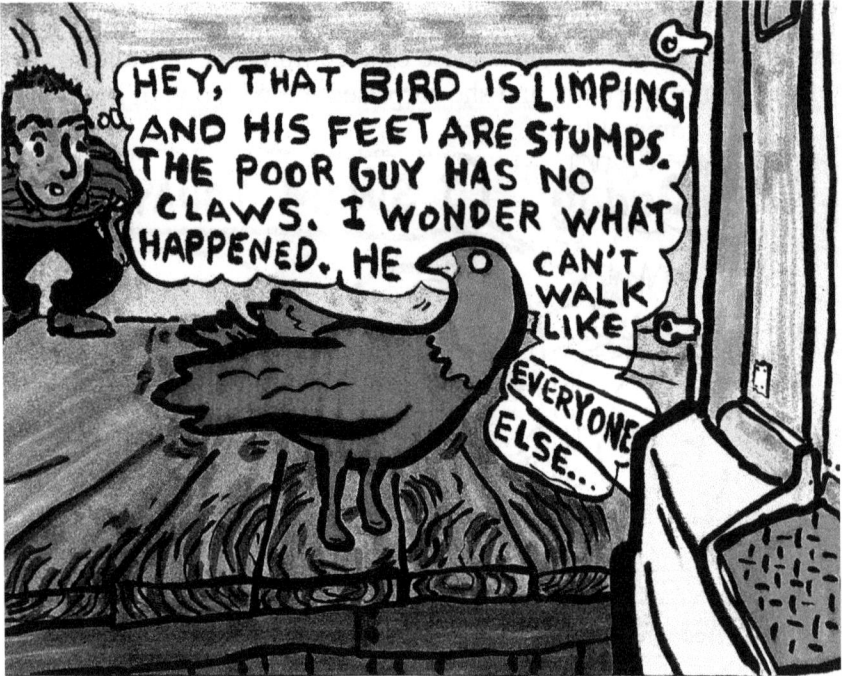

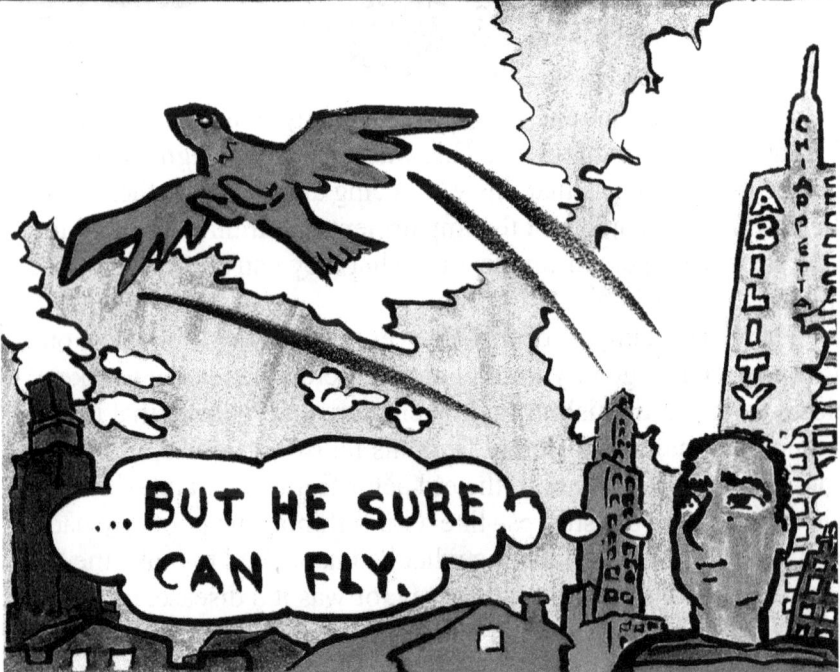

When that same bird suddenly took flight like a champion through the sky faster than I could even process a feeble thought, I fumbled to amend my flawed analysis. No getting around it; I was wrong about the bird's ability--dead wrong.

I think this bird was a pigeon. When he flew away, it half surprised me that he could maneuver in the air just like the other birds. Then I realized that this was prejudicial thinking on my part, and that is exactly what people do to people with disabilities--much of the time. Just because a person doesn't have a particular ability in one area, doesn't mean that the whole person is broken through and through. This is something to be remembered. Disabled or not, all people have some sort of unique ability.

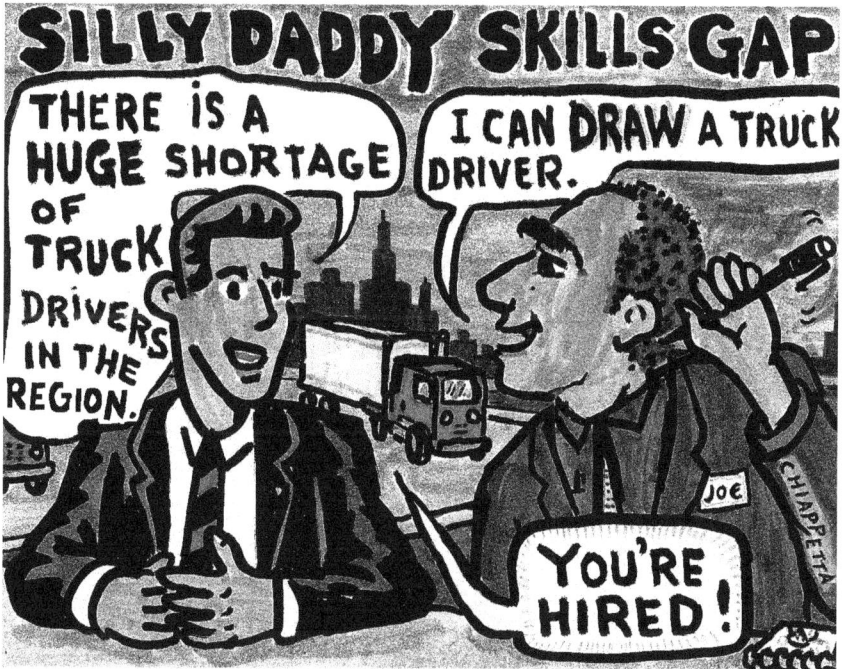

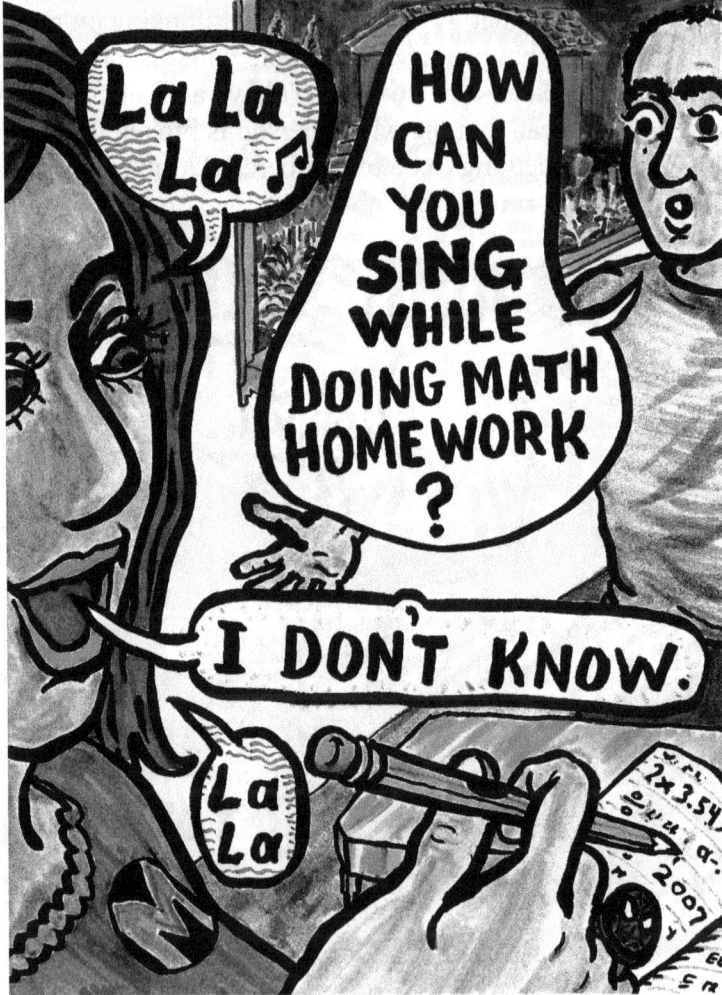

Chapter 10:

Ramping Up to Be Healed

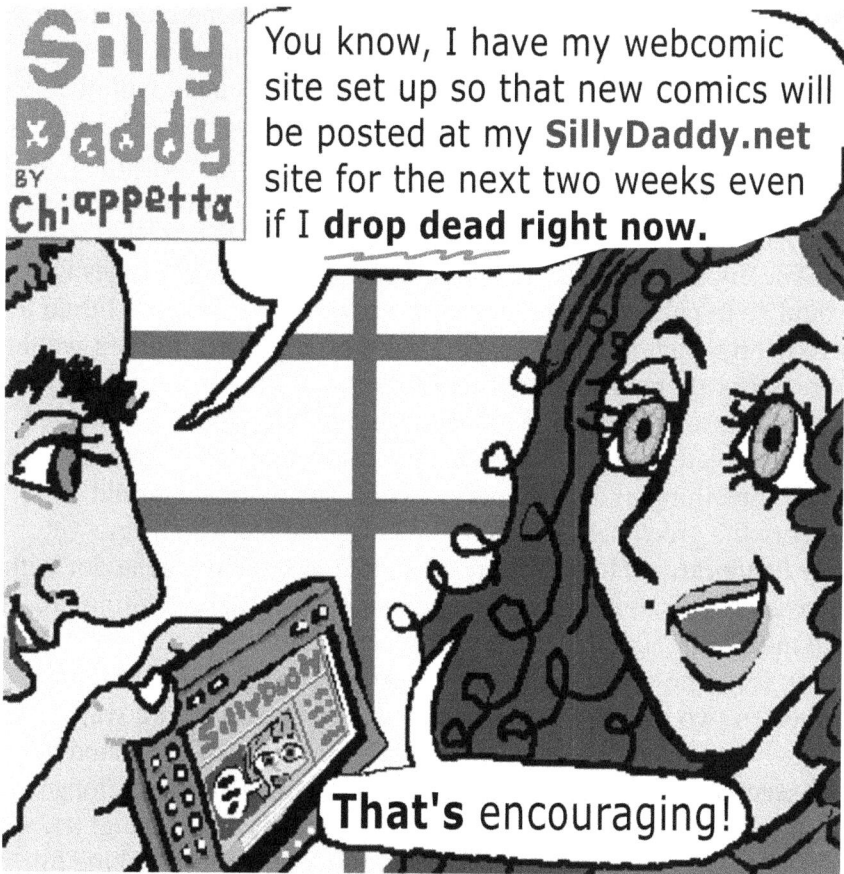

Despite all the quick fixes and temporary work-arounds that I had discovered to alleviate some of my back pain, I could not be satisfied with a little relief. Sometimes I would get sad and even weirdly morbid at the thought of prolonged living in a state of discomfort and only partial recovery. This can be evident in the bizarre conversation I had with Silly Sister while I was boasting, as if I had something to boast about.

Shortly after accomplishing my task of being "two weeks into the future" with my online comics publishing, I realized the futility of it. Ecclesiastes 9:5 declares that the memory of the dead will be forgotten. I had to face the facts; no matter how many weeks into the "future" I schedule my comics blog, I'll still eventually die at some point, so why not live life to the full now. It's what I do while I am alive that matters. Comics can't truly extend my life or heal anyone-- only God can do that. Why shouldn't I believe that God can completely make me new again? He's God after all.

Therefore, I wanted the complete fix--total regeneration. Fellow back pain-suffering folks will be relieved and/or amazed to know that just a few months after my "broken robot" moment with the green ball and Silly Sister, I became completely healed of back pain, which had plagued me for most of my adult life. How I came to be healed is a tale filled with mysteries, clues, faith, action, and repentance.

The mysteries had to do with the few, but refreshing times I would be in pain one minute, yet the next, be fine for a bit. I tried to zero in on which factors impacted those brief periods where I would be temporarily pain-free. At first it was just a mystery. Justin, my personal trainer, pointed me in the right direction, but I still longed to be completely rid of this back pain. I now knew, as Justin did, that it had something to do with nerves, because any time I would squeeze the green ball, the pain would immediately go away--yet only temporarily. However, once I started to track my behavior with increased focus, more patterns emerged. The clues kept piling up, like mud on a rainy day: messy and unavoidable.

In fact, one such pile of clues happened shortly after a big rain. I had taken two of my kids to a nearby forest preserve for a walk through the fields. We came upon a great expanse of open land that just seemed like a special place to get some fresh air after a long winter. With my seven-year-old son and three-year-old daughter, we crossed a grassy clearing until it gave way to a modest looking hill where there used to be an old stone quarry. That particular day, the area was simply covered thoroughly with the blackest of mud, which to my explorer's eyes seemed to be the perfect place to walk up and have a look about from on high.

That the mud was quite wet and sticky did not at first appear to be a big deal. We all had our toughest waterproof boots on, so what harm could a little muddy hill do to us? More than meets the eye, I soon found out. The first sign of trouble occurred when my daughter said, "My feet keep getting stuck in this mud. Carry me, Daddy! Carry me, carry me." As if to further illustrate her point, Anna's little pink boot got stuck in the mud and her foot popped out. Instinctively, I swiftly picked her up so that she wouldn't fall sideways into the muddy slope, and was surprised to discover that my back wasn't burning in agony. My son Luke was slowly trudging ahead of us, so I called out to him, "Son, try to find the driest route to the top of the hill!"

Luke did so, and I decided to boldly carry Anna up the muddy slope. However, I started to feel an increase to my back pain. If it were any other situation, I would have naturally put Anna back down and said, "Sorry, my back is messed up. I can't carry you. You're going to have to walk yourself." Yet since I did not want my child wriggling about in the mud, clamoring for a way home like some wild animal, this was not an option. I had to figure out a way to keep carrying my daughter. She was counting on it. Therefore, I squeezed my knees together as if an imaginary green ball was between my legs. This in turn forced my lower back muscles to relax and the pain in my spine would go away for a few minutes.

In this way, we slowly climbed up that muddy hill, but then my own feet got stuck, and I mean completely stuck. All the while I was holding Anna, and everywhere I turned to try and walk, I would just keep getting stuck as my feet sunk deeper and deeper into the ground. By this point, Anna was afraid to be let back down, and I don't blame her. So I held her while we prayed for a way out of this muddy mess.

We may have been stuck there indefinitely, had it not been for my trusty son Luke. No one else was there to witness our pathetic little muddy hike, so help had to come from our own dwindling might and wits. Gratefully, my son went and gathered rocks for me to step on. I literally had to walk on a makeshift path he laid out of random stones. After thirty minutes of this, we finally made it back to grassy ground. Exhausted, I put Anna down and learned two valuable things on that bizarre expedition: walking up muddy hills was a terrible idea, and more importantly, my back was much stronger than I thought it was.

I believe that God got a big kick out of seeing us through that situation, and not just because of how ridiculous we must have looked, being stuck in the mud and unable to move more than one foot every minute or so. In Psalm 37:23, it says, **"If the LORD delights in a man's way, he makes his steps firm; though he stumble, he will not fall, for the LORD upholds him with his hand."**

Despite my foolishness for leading the family into such difficult terrain, my belief is that God delighted in the fact that I was finally showing some courage. This was probably the longest time I had ever held my daughter in a standing position. That took courage, because I had been so afraid of lifting anything for years. Though I stumbled and stalled often through that muddy slope, God upheld us with his mighty hand. I began to understand that pleasing God could be so intricately connected with healing. Naturally, from this point forward, I was inspired to increase my courage and please God even more.

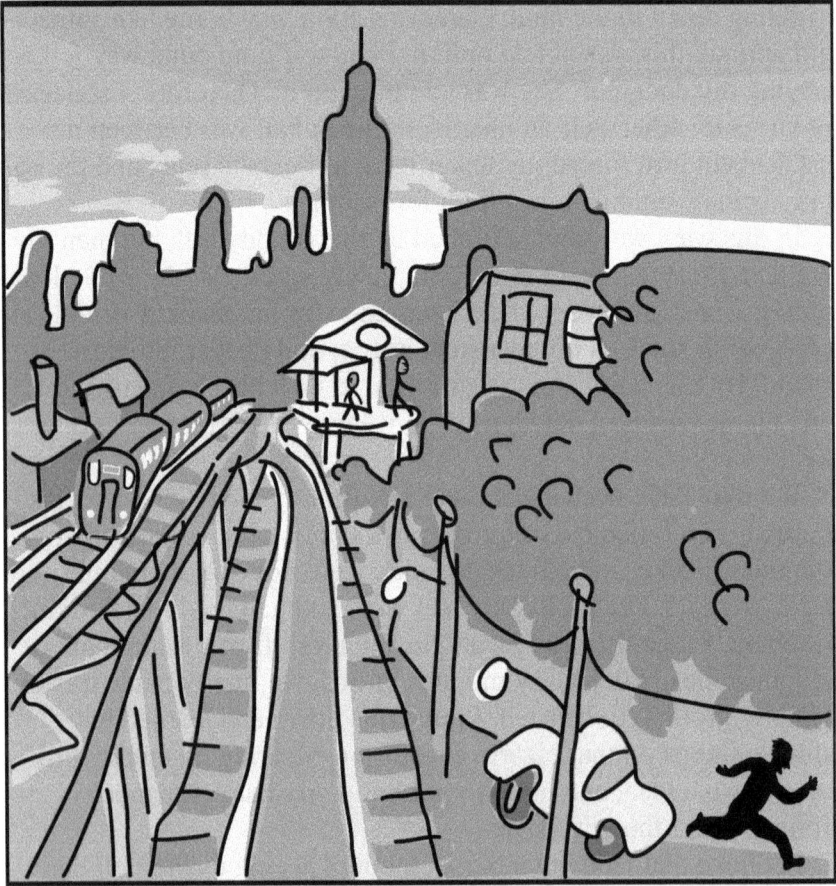

Another clue to what was going on with my back was hidden in a number of seemingly unrelated activities. Whenever I felt claustrophobic from being on a bus or a train for too long, and then got off and ran home for a few blocks, I would experience no pain in my lower back while running. Whenever I would sing tenor with the church and it was a complex harmonic song I really got into, like "I'll Fly Away," my back pain would mysteriously disappear for the entire song. Whenever I was sitting in a Bible study with someone who wanted to learn about becoming a Christian, and I had to make an important point that involved expressing something very deep, I was (you guessed it) pain-free for that period.

If I hadn't made note of the claustrophobic bus and train-running scenarios, I might think that it was simply a case of God giving me relief during times of intense spiritual focus. However, there is nothing at all spiritual about running away from a bus because I couldn't stand to be around so many people anymore. So what was the common thread in all of these activities? Only later I would come to understand that it was the sense of single-minded freedom and guilt-free gratification that allowed me to experience pain relief.

First, however, I had to go through something I like to think of as the flat tire test. As a parent, I'm always trying to teach my kids one thing or another to live by. Therefore, it should come as no surprise that God, as my father, was teaching me something to live by as well. Apparently, though, I needed a lot of practice before I could fully get it.

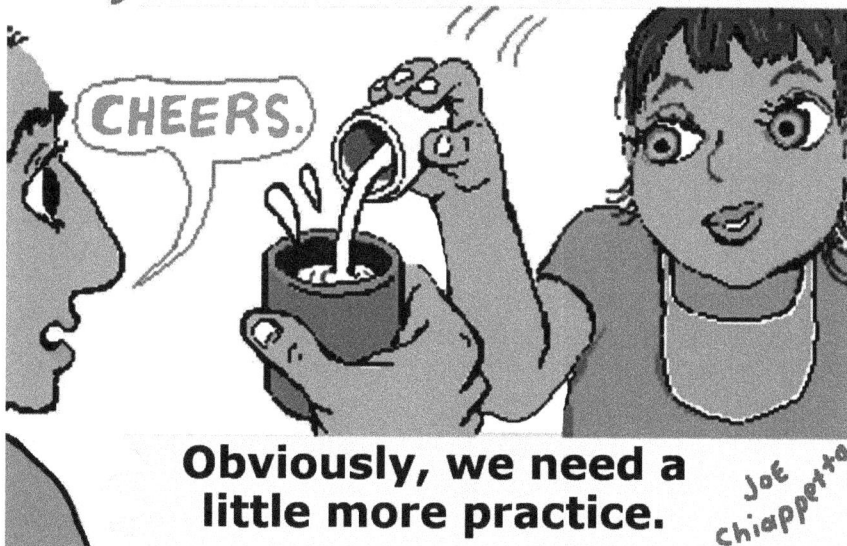

Silly Daddy

I'm teaching my daughter how to make a toast.

CHEERS.

Obviously, we need a little more practice.

Joe Chiappetta

Chapter 11:

The Flat Tire Test

My friend Jay and I were talking about the correlation between faith and my back injury one day, and he picked up on something that I was lacking. So he said this; "You know, Jesus says that if you have faith and do not doubt, you can say to this mountain 'go throw yourself into the sea,' and it will be done! What you have to understand, Joe, is that his statement is either true or it's a lie. If you believe the scriptures, and I know you do, then you need to increase your faith about being healed. Do you believe that Jesus has the power to heal you?"

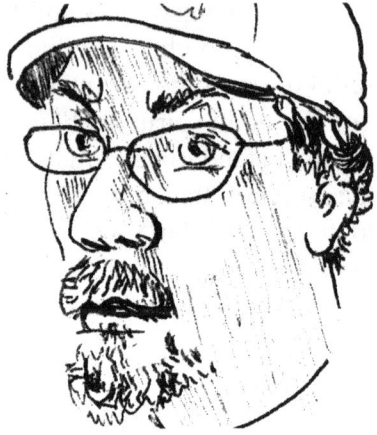

I thought for quite some time about this conversation. I had been praying about being healed for so very long, yet did I really believe that complete healing was in store for me? Had my doubts been a deterrent to the healing touch of God? I suspected that they were, so I had to step out on faith about this issue. Some sort of decisive action was needed on my part, to put my faith and deeds on the same playing field.

One evening, after a long and painful day, I prayed, "God, please put me in a situation where I would normally say 'No' to a physical activity involving my back. But this time, when you put me in such a physically demanding position, let me say 'Yes' to it. Then let me go and do whatever that activity is and be healed by it."

What I had in mind was perhaps someone who was moving would ask me to help them lift a lot of boxes, or some other strenuous life situation that I had almost always said "No" to over the years because of my back. Not five minutes after I had prayed this prayer, I got a call from a friend of the family.

She said, "Sorry to bother you, but my tire gave out on my car and I am a few blocks from your house. Can you help me fix a flat?"

It actually started to rain as I ran to the rescue. I immediately knew that God had answered my prayer. Not aware of my prayer, however, my wife tried to stop me. "You can't go out there!" she said with fear. "You'll make yourself even worse!"

"Honey," I replied, understanding that her fears were the same captivating fears that I had been a slave to for so long, "don't worry about it. I have to do this. It is an answer to my prayers. God is going to heal me through this."

I didn't wait for further objections. I went into the rain and fixed that flat--jacking up the car, lifting off one tire, putting on the spare--all without an ounce of pain. It was amazing. It was the power of God!

Halfway through the flat-fixing, my friend said, "Oh, wait, I forgot about your bad back--I shouldn't have called you! I'm so sorry."

"No need to apologize," I replied with the confidence of a superhero. "God himself has allowed me to fix your flat tire!"

I thought this victory over fear would be the complete end of my back pain. However, a few days later, I had reverted to my old, painful self again, complete with lower lumbar aches and pains that ceased to go away. What was going on here? I had a taste of the glory--but now it was gone. I wondered if it was gone for good. The thought of living with this lower back issue for the rest of my life was most discouraging.

I was swimming multiple times a week, working out with the green ball every morning, increasing my faith, and facing my fears. What else was left to do? Quite a bit, as it turned out. I believe all this time, God was asking me, "Who are you really relying on, me or yourself?"

As previously mentioned, I had seen a slew of medical professionals about my back over the years. To this day, I am still asking, "Why?" I sum up all those healthcare visits with an imaginary scenario where I'm wired up in a doctor's office, shackled to the latest overpriced gizmo that claims to cure back pain. No matter how confident or respectful the doctor sounds, I flash back to that helpless feeling I encountered in the hospital while visiting a dear member of my family. Whether these characters could heal me or not, being at the mercy of doctors was so unsettling. The only thing I could be sure of was that my life was certainly not in my hands, and that didn't sit well with me. Yet why should I be surprised? After all, sitting was a major part of the problem.

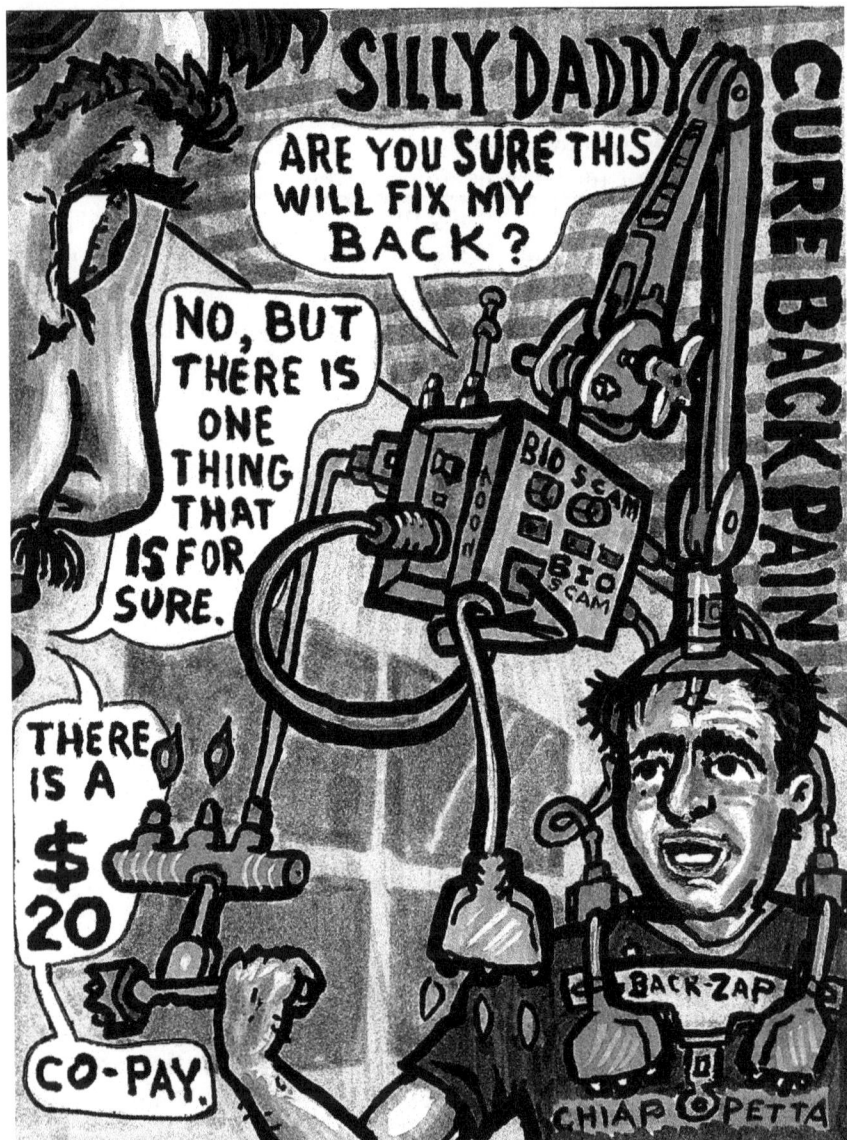

I started to wonder if there would ever be an independence day from the daily grind of chronic back pain. Only the makers of the Bio-Scam Back Zap gizmo know for sure.

Most people who have back pain or health insurance might appreciate this joke. It's so funny, it hurts--or maybe it just plain hurts.

Medical costs were starting to add up. The more I paid for them, the more I realized that these medical professionals were just guessing at what was wrong. They were taking shots in the dark. I spent so much down time in quiet waiting rooms, that I began to wonder if God just wanted me to have some more moments to meditate on my life and on his mighty deeds. Sitting around for so long doing nothing in a doctor's office would also occasionally yield more than a few bizarre ideas--my own meaningless shots in the dark.

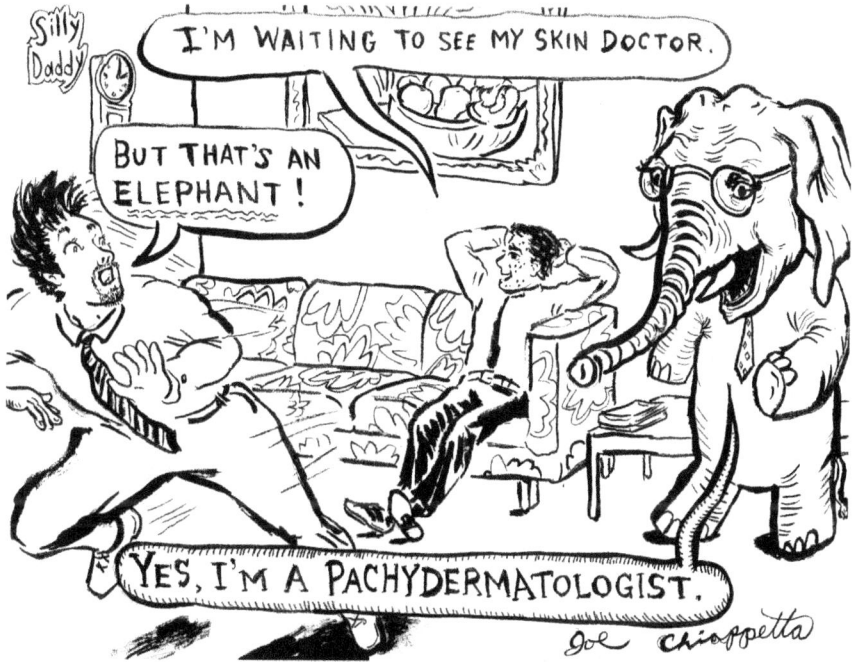

Wasn't there anyone on this earth to rescue me? I kept waiting for my Back Pain Avenger, but no one took on the role. It was so frustrating; the most help I received was from people who had no medical degrees, namely Justin, the personal trainer, and Jay, the Christian who challenged my faith. The last medical professionals I went to see were in the most respected healthcare job of them all: that of a surgeon. After a two-minute conversation, one surgeon showed me a hard plastic device that would be surgically implanted into my spine and screwed in place. That was quite horrifying! It was about the size of a hockey puck. All I had to do was sign some papers and a surgery date would be set. Something in my gut told me that this surgical procedure called "lumbar fusion" was not a good idea.

Therefore, I got another opinion from a different surgeon. He spent less than one minute with me, asked me only one question, and then told me when he was available to do the surgery. Something was not right. This was just too easy. I decided to read up on spinal fusion surgery, and am so glad I did. In everything I read, the patients aren't really healed, and rather are more prone to have the same procedure done on another part of their back later in life. This was progress? I think not. Where was the Back Pain Avenger when I needed him most? Did he even exist, or was complete healing just a figment of my imagination? If the Back Pain Avenger did exist, surely now, surrounded by so many misleading doctors, would be a good time to appear. Avenge me, please, from the hands of these overpriced and ill-equipped professionals. Back Pain Avenger, come quickly!

Someone reminded me of the woman from the fifth chapter of Mark. She was subject to bleeding for twelve years, and no one could heal her. In fact, the Bible says that the situation was extremely dire:

"She had suffered a great deal under the care of many doctors and had spent all she had, yet instead of getting better, she grew worse."

Finally, when she came close to Jesus and touched his cloak, she had faith that this would heal her. And it did!

I kept praying that God would make it clear what I should do about my own situation, because I really was running out of patience. Did I need to get closer to Jesus, like the bleeding woman, whom no one else could heal? I didn't know how much longer I could operate at such a constant level of discomfort. Yet the bleeding woman did not let her pain stop her from getting closer to Jesus. Could I say the same?

Aggressively working on increasing my faith in Christ became a constant focus--not just a one-day flat tire fix. This attitude prepared me for the next and final step in the healing process. The element that pushed me over the top into complete healing was reading and applying the principles in a book called *Healing Back Pain: The Mind-Body Connection*, by John E. Sarno, MD. Ironically, someone in the swimming pool locker room recommended this exact book to me a year prior, but I ignored their input. Gratefully, a coworker named Lance later gave this book to me--he put it in my hands and said, "This is for you." However, I still didn't read it right away. I had my wife--a very fast reader--go through it first. She tore through it with amazement and said, "Joseph, this book has you totally pegged! Read it, like immediately."

Finally, I complied, and quickly discovered that it's a book the spinal fusion surgery-loving medical establishment doesn't want you to read. But don't let that stop you. The book indeed described my situation exactly, although at first I didn't want to admit it. There were tons of deep, emotional issues I had refused to deal with over the years. The brain has to do something with all that unresolved pain. Since the mind doesn't want to express this pain, the brain re-routes the stress of the issue down the nerves to another area of the body. For me, that was my lower back, the bearer of all sorts of complex emotions that I was too cowardly to deal with in my mind over the years.

Once I accepted this, I started repenting. An attitude of complete openness was adopted, and I dug up uncomfortable emotional issues that had plagued me for too long. I prayed about these hurts, and had hard talks with the people I needed to, with long overdue tears. Humiliating as it is to admit, here are some of the key issues I had to dig up, expose, and face head-on:

My Sobering Six Statements

1) I was ashamed of my failures in parenting.

2) I was fearful of getting older and losing more abilities.

3) I was disappointed with God and myself over the limited success of my creative career as an artist and a writer.

4) I was mad at myself for not studying a more practical career track in college.

5) I was sorrowful over all the pain I had caused my family over the years, due to my own arrogance.

6) I was deceitful. Despite my reputation for being a smiling Silly Daddy, I wasn't always happy.

These were my six shameful truths. Unsettling as they were, like a long overdue bout of tears, it was good to get them out in the open. Within a few days after I read Sarno's book, I faced my failures (also known as my sin) and attempted to understand these issues from a spiritual point of view. Thereafter--I kid you not--I was completely pain-free! Why? Because I had gotten open, confessed these sins to

God and man, and repented. The scripture about confession that was applied here is from James 5:16.

"Therefore, confess your sins to each other and pray for each other so that you may be healed. The prayer of a righteous person is powerful and effective."

That phrase "so that you may be healed," shows the conditional aspects of the healing process. Simply praying and confessing to God is not enough here. "Righteous" followers of Jesus must be directly involved. Therefore, I followed this biblical pattern in a non-fragmented manner. All in the same week, I confessed to other disciples of Jesus, prayed with them, and applied the will of God, also known as righteousness, to my life. A careful study of this verse reveals the life-altering connection between confession (to faithful followers of Jesus) and healing (through prayer).

A mild disclaimer is in order at this point regarding Sarno's book, *Healing Back Pain*. Matters of healing and God might be obvious to followers of Jesus, but not so clear to people who are fuzzy about their faith. I am certain that many people, looking for a shortcut, will simply try to read Sarno's book and think that's enough to be healed. In fact, if I were not a follower of Jesus, that is exactly what I would do. For me, however, that would fall incredibly short. In fact, I had read an earlier book by Sarno on the same topic over a decade prior, yet it had no healing impact in my life. While Sarno's *Healing Back Pain* book was incredibly helpful, I cannot emphasize enough the following reality; it was my active faith in Jesus, combined with true understanding, which led me to radical sweeping repentance. My belief is that these elements--faith, truth, and repentance--worked together to inspire God to bring me complete healing.

I'm not saying not to go and read Sarno's book. His work guided me greatly to get to the full truth quicker. Sarno helped me with the understanding element. Moreover, if I ever met John Sarno, I would give him a giant hug, and perhaps even lift him off the ground as a sign of gratitude. That said, the greater glory goes to God, who makes everything new.

Finally, what could only be the work of the Back Pain Avenger was shown in fullness; he had saved the day. For years--decades even--I had almost given up on complete healing, yet that was to my shame. It was always Jesus who saves. **"It is mine to avenge,"** says the Lord. (Romans 12:19)

I think back to my moments of darkest despair and realize, to my shame, that the main hindrance to my being rescued was always me.

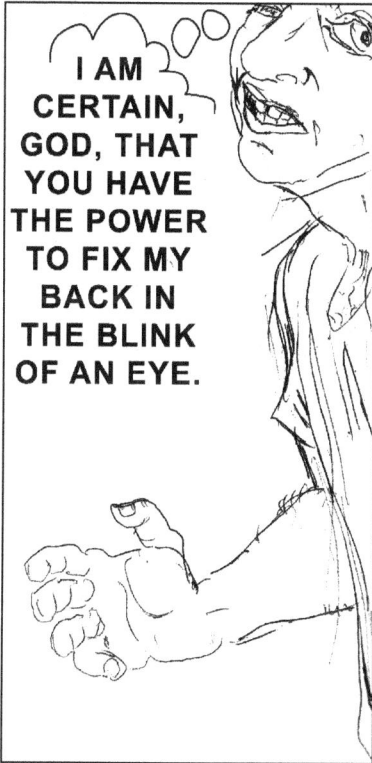

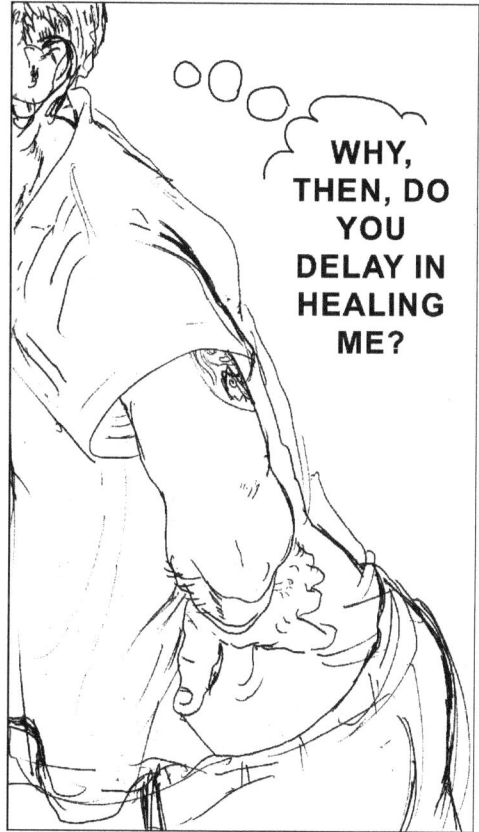

The problem wasn't God, the government, my spouse, my kids, my job, the economy, or any of that stuff. The problem was always me. As soon as my sin got out of the way, and my faith turned into high gear, that's when God did his thing. He showed up right in time, as my Back Pain Avenger.

Chapter 12:

Captain Disability to the Rescue?

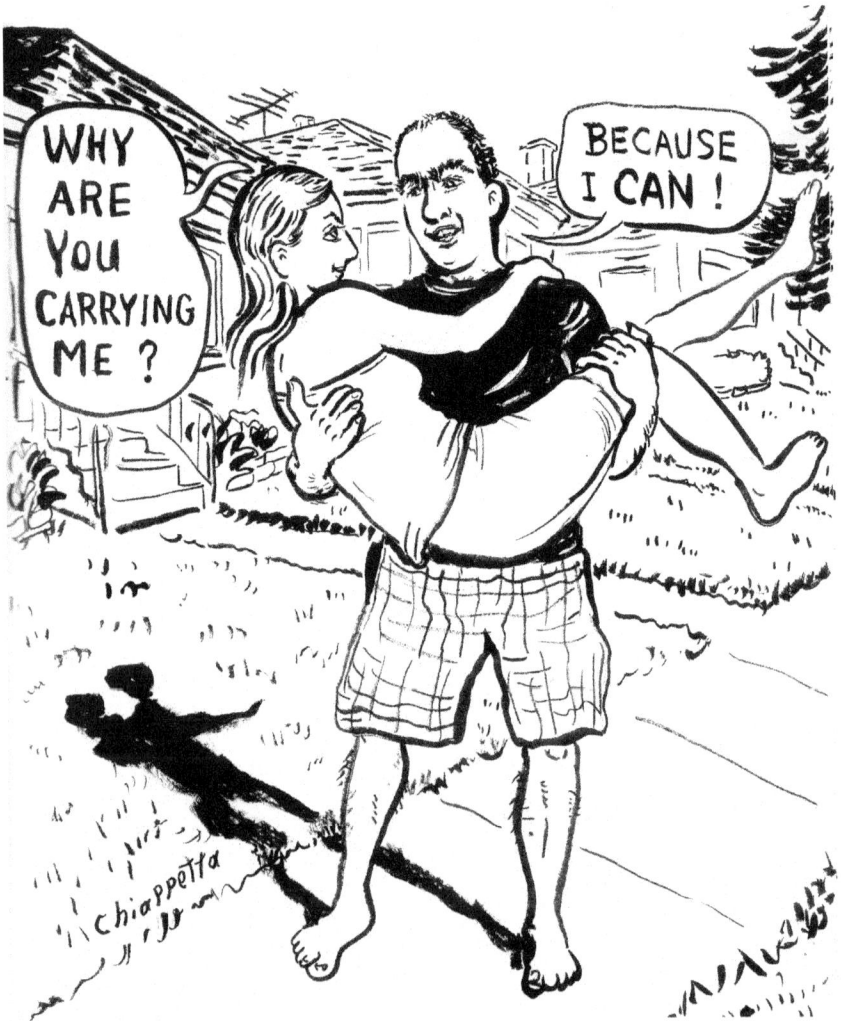

Once I realized that my pain had been avenged and I was my own worst enemy, I started to tell all sorts of people the changes that I was going through, and what had made me well again. For heightened drama, when reaching the climax in the story of how I got healed, I would often pick up my wife completely off the ground and gently toss her in the air. Catching her steadily seemed like the most direct way to demonstrate the complete transformation I had gone through: from a man afraid to pick up a baby to a man flinging his wife into the air. I felt this scripture from Psalm 30:2-3 come alive even more:

"O LORD, my God, I called to you for help and you healed me. O LORD, you brought me up from the grave; you spared me from going down into the pit."

I was so blown away by what God had done with my life that, out of sheer joy, sometimes I would pick up Denise even when there was no one around to hear my amazing story. With curious surprise, my wife would ask, "What are you doing? Why are you carrying me?"

With the confidence of a champion/barbarian, I would reply, "Because I can!"

I was also able to carry my little ones as needed once again. This was something I hadn't regularly done in years! Life was renewed, and as a family, we took trips to the woods and built little forts for fun. Once, while all five of us were traveling through the forest, I jokingly said to my youngest daughter as I held her, "Soon, you'll be too big for me to carry you."

Since this particular hike took longer than usual, and we were traveling along a trail that we had not taken all together, my oldest daughter asked, "What are we even doing out here?"

As we approached our crude, yet lovable little hut made out of sticks, I explained, "Your brother and I built a fort in the forest. We're downsizing."

Noticing the low ceiling of the fort, my youngest daughter yelled out in objection, "We can't downsize! I'm still growing."

We often joke about what it might be like if we actually lived in a muddy fort in the woods. I typically view such outings as an instant getaway--a free vacation. However, I might be in the minority. My youngest daughter put things into perspective when she was praying one night. After a long day playing at the fort, she closed her conversation with God by adding, "And God, thank you that we could go to the fort and have some fun. But thank you that we don't have to live in the fort, and thank you that we can sleep in a nice warm house in a nice warm bed."

What else can you say to that but "Amen"?

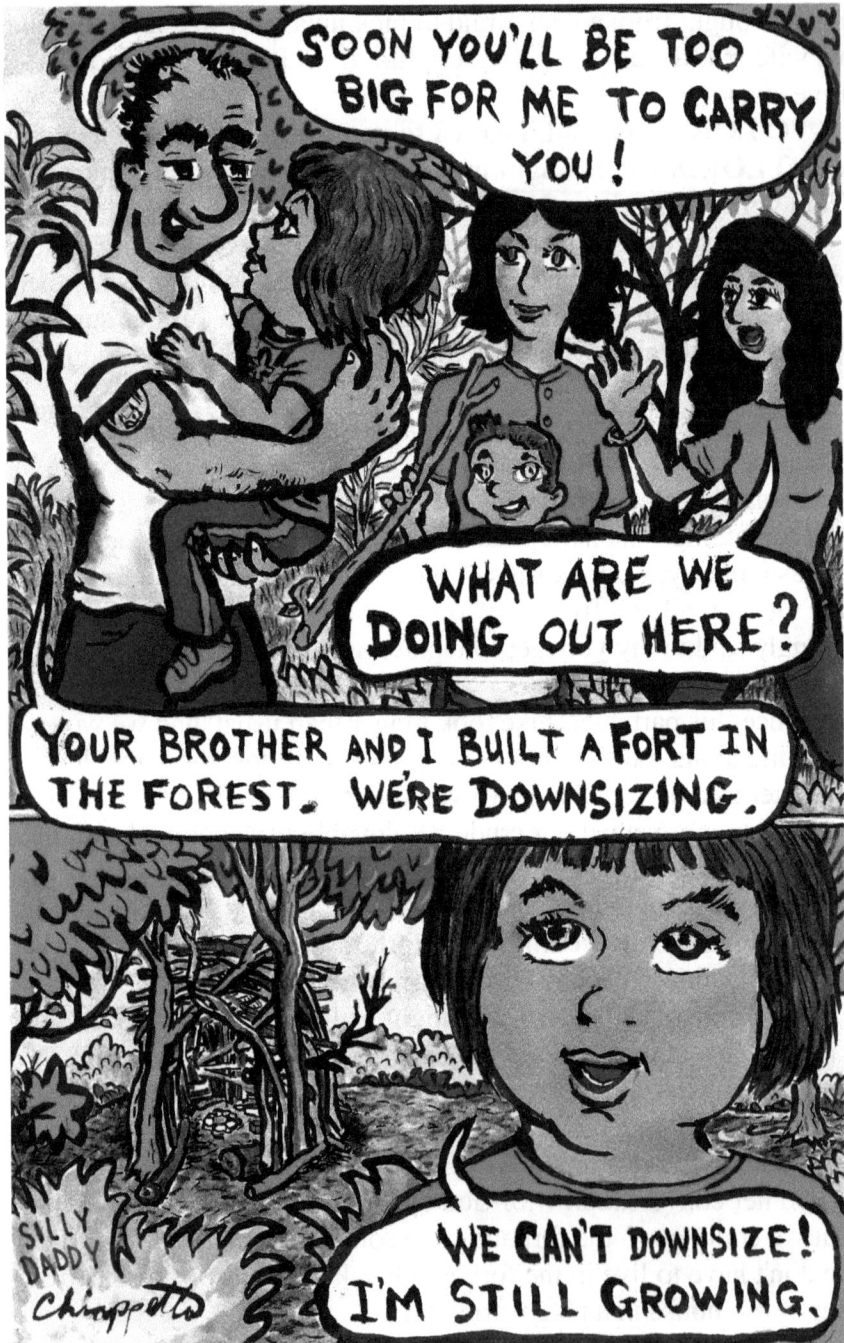

It was around this time when the fort-building and random wife-lifting heroics began that Denise and a number of other friends gave me career-specific advice that I never imagined ever following. They consistently started to urge me to write about my experience with disability more purposefully. I shrugged off these suggestions for quite some time. I was free of that troublesome period of my life; why would I want to relive it?

The answer to that question kept creeping up on me. Either I never noticed it before, or the encounters were increasing, but I kept running into more and more people who were in the middle of similar chronic back pain issues. The more I learned about the chronic pain of others, the more I started to identify non-coincidental parallels with my own situation. Perhaps I had something to offer them.

People, especially those in the midst of their chronic pains, asked me with heightened interest, "How did you get healed? I need to know." Thereafter, I would make attempts to explain the whole amazing ordeal, but for time's sake, I would always leave various details out, or simply forget them. Of course, whenever I would tell them as much as I could remember in one sitting, those in the depths of their own pain would always light up with hope, as in, "If it worked for you, it could work for me." I began to see how important the fine details of my story had become. For many, my story could mean the difference between regeneration and degeneration.

What put me over the top and made me commit to writing the account of how I got healed was something my wife said. She had just finished reading my sequel to *Star Chosen*, which is a science fiction book entitled *Power Pendant of Planet Pizon*. Being the first person to read the book before I published it, I was certainly very eager to hear what she thought.

The first book had been very well received, and I had taken a slightly different approach with the second book: more action, more romance, and a major character gets killed. Naturally, I wanted to make sure I was going in the right direction, and Denise, in addition to being a great writer and editor, has a knack for knowing when I'm onto something, and when I'm not.

"So, what do you think?" I asked her, almost impatiently. Surely she would see the genius in my space-romance-gone-bad story that involves a fight over a high-tech triangular pendant that draws its power only from pure spiritual strength. Surely she would be on the edge of her seat screaming "live long and prosper!" as well as crying for an encore and anticipating the day when my *Star Chosen* series would take its rightful place next to the *John Carter, Warlord of Mars* series.

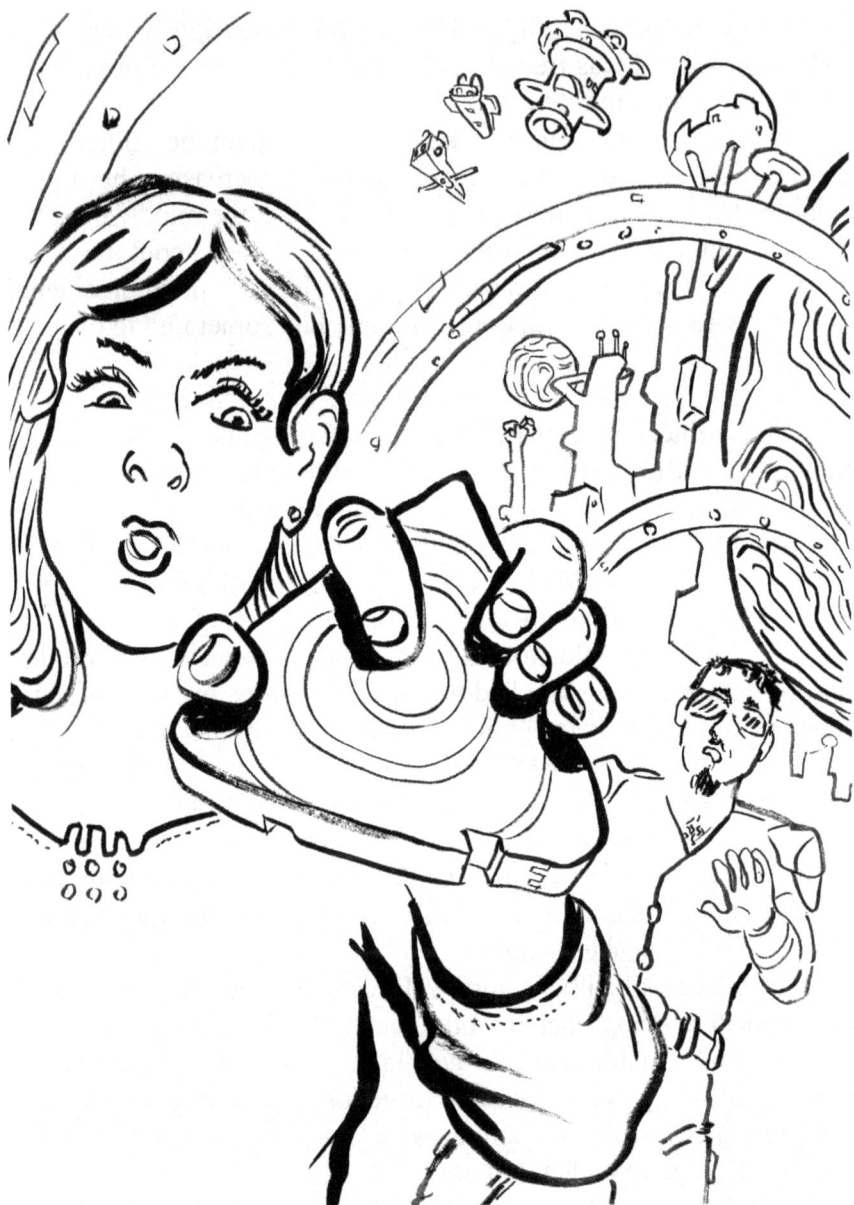

After all this grandiose anticipation, my wife said to me, "Joseph, don't get me wrong--the story is very good--it's solid science fiction. But I still think you need to write a disability book. I mean, I know you spend a lot of your creative time on the comics and the science fiction novels, and sure, you can do that. Yet look at what you've been through. I think God has set you up to write your disability story so that people can benefit from it."

Always the quick study, I asked, "What are you talking about? I've been doing comics since the late 1980s and writing science fiction off and on for over a decade. How does disability fit in?"

With complete sureness, Denise replied, "How many other experienced writers do you know that have lived with a disability, have been cured of that disability, and have been working in the disability field for the past ten years like you? Who else has all those traits?"

"Well, no one that I know of," I sheepishly answered. Why, oh why does she always have to be right?

"That's my whole point," Denise replied. "I believe that God has prepared you for this book--a disability book. I mean, you are the leader of the oldest disability-focused workforce developer network in Chicago. Leaders lead and write about it. This is the book you should write."

"Aw, what does she know anyways? She doesn't even read science fiction unless I write it. Why am I even asking her? She's a nonfiction fan. Where are my sci-fi geek buddies when I need them?" These were my first thoughts, not that I said them out loud.

Nevertheless, the more I thought about it, the more I realized that she was right. Leaders lead. If they don't, they cease to be true leaders. The reason I was initially so resistant to the idea of writing completely about my disability was really quite simple. I didn't want to write about it because that would be hard work: digging up the sorry degradation of my mortality and trying to make sense of it in a larger context. Yet isn't that part of what leaders do from time to time, blazing the uncharted trail in search of the greater good? Wait, isn't that what leaders do all the time?

How could I also forget that leaders work hard? Was I afraid of hard work? If so, it was time to face my fears, since *not* facing fears was part of what sunk me deeper into chronic health problems in the first place.

In light of my wife's very fine exhortation, once her urging sunk in, I wasted no time in coming up with the most fun part of writing a book: thinking up cool names for the title. A few days later, I thanked my wife and resolutely set out to do exactly what she was advising. I was officially on board.

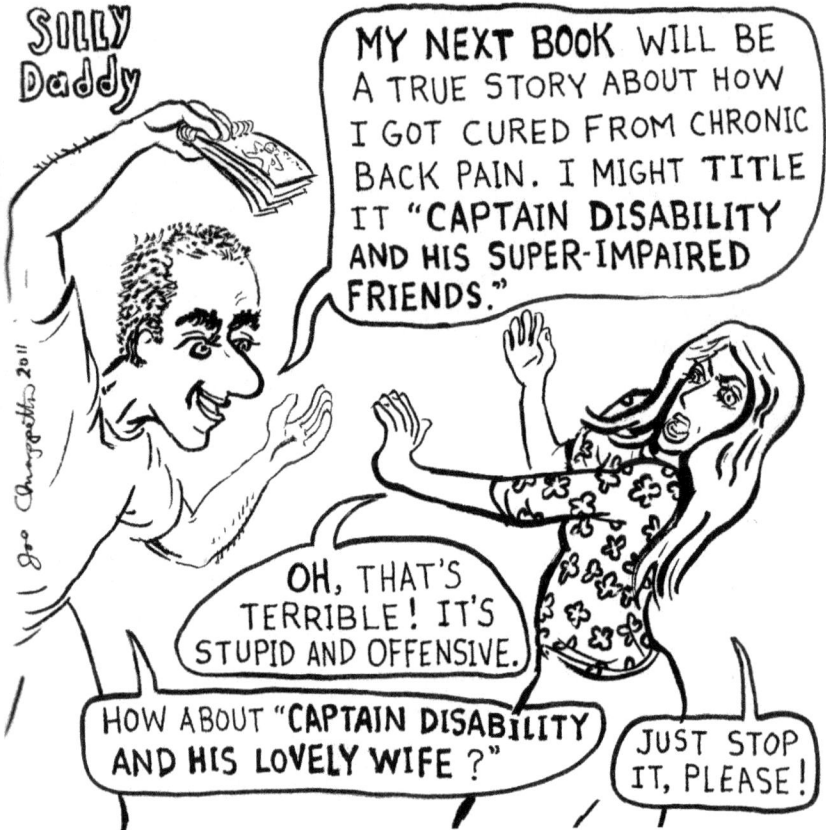

SILLY Daddy

MY NEXT BOOK WILL BE A TRUE STORY ABOUT HOW I GOT CURED FROM CHRONIC BACK PAIN. I MIGHT TITLE IT "CAPTAIN DISABILITY AND HIS SUPER-IMPAIRED FRIENDS."

OH, THAT'S TERRIBLE! IT'S STUPID AND OFFENSIVE.

HOW ABOUT "CAPTAIN DISABILITY AND HIS LOVELY WIFE?"

JUST STOP IT, PLEASE!

This was a real conversation that we had, and all kidding aside, I am so very grateful to Denise and her ability to see God's hand in my disability recovery, as well as his influence in my creative endeavors. From then on, I saw all sorts of things God had allowed to happen that could be used in my first book completely focused on disability issues.

I was actually alarmed to realize the large amount of cartoons I had drawn over the years which made reference to my back pain. Prior to my wife spurring me into this topic, I just assumed I hardly wrote about it much, if even at all. Yet the opposite is true. Disability was on my mind all these years as a topic that subconsciously populated an increasing number of my *Silly Daddy* comics. If disability matters got into my work subconsciously, I wondered what I might create if I focused on it intentionally.

This was a turning point for me. It made it easier to embrace my role as a leader in the disability community, as a writer, and as a man following God. Often I see these duties as completely separate, yet I don't think God sees it as such. Perhaps for the first time ever, I got a glimpse of how those roles are all tied together, and I could use them to help inspire others. God, the Back Pain Avenger, strikes again!

Surely God works through many people to inspire us. I now specifically believed that it was time for him to work through me.

Chapter 13: Unbearable Troubles

(Nothing New Yet No Less Dramatic)

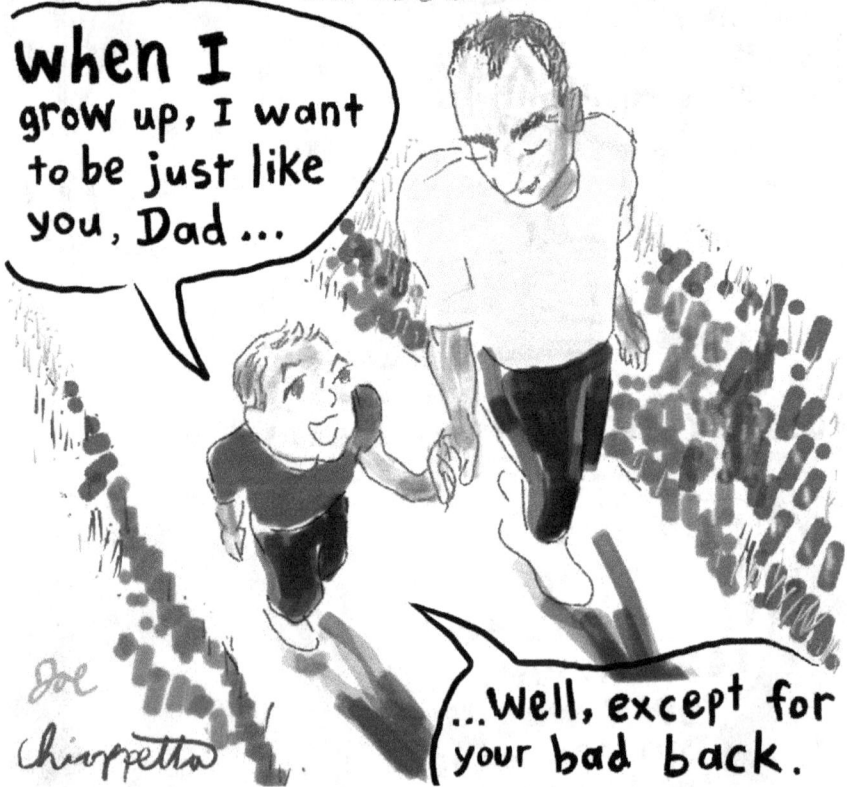

Spiritual matters play such a huge role in disability matters. I have seen this professionally and personally. When I am focused on God and am prayerful about my role to help people with disabilities through the workforce developer network, I have always found that this is when the most job placements occur.

Moreover, on an even more personal level, it's the only way I survived through what I thought were times of unbearable pain due to my own lower back injury. I dreamed to be free of this burden for a long, long time. In fact, the pain was something I had struggled with for 25 years--more than half of my life! My son, for the first eight years of his life, just took it as normal for his dad to have a disability.

There were times--faithless times--when I just assumed that I would be stuck with this pain for the rest of my life. My son making such a matter-of-fact statement was very telling. It revealed a lot about my own behavior that needed to change. Of course, I'm glad that he wanted to be like me, but the fact that he so blatantly identified me with my back pain showed how much of my life revolved around my disability. That simply had to stop. It was a wake-up call for me to say no to functional limitations prescribed by doctors.

I am so glad that I didn't stay in a mental state consumed by my own disability. That was another key element in my rehabilitation process. I had to stop living in fear of making my back pain worse. I had to start living my life again, and step out on faith. Now, thanks to God, my lower back injury is gone and I can dart about like a squirrel again. Without faith, this never would have happened.

The reason that the seemingly unbearable situation of my back injury has been on my mind more and more lately is because I have two friends in prison. I will only touch on the fact that both of them also have a disability. Researchers who are better equipped than I am can go on and on about how too many people with disabilities end up in jail, partly because social support systems failed them, or misunderstood them early on.

When I even try to consider the predicament of my two jailed friends, I fall completely short of understanding, even though I have had my bouts with the unbearable. Some of the terrible things they tell me in their letters about prison life seem to be completely beyond my imagination. What can I do for them? Certainly I can pray--and I do. Yet how do I communicate with them in a way that connects? Is empathy even possible? Perhaps thinking about what got me through the back pain will somehow create a point of relatability that clicks with my imprisoned friends. Therefore, I must reflect upon what got me through the unbearable periods in my life. The answer comes quickly and without question: it is God.

In times of unbearable trouble, it is important to search for the presence of God working through the situation. That is how I survived my back injury and am now completely healed. Most of what God was doing, even in the beginning of the pain, I was oblivious to. It literally took decades for me to understand what God was trying to show me. And until I was ready to comprehend the lesson and apply it to my life, the pain would continue, since God disciplines those he loves, as the book of Hebrews explains in sobering detail. The lesson was that I needed to change my character with a complete overhaul. I needed humility, sincerity, deeper faith and openness.

While this book is a fairly detailed account of how I was healed, the one thing I should stress about the whole draining ordeal is this: once I dealt with the issues God wanted me to deal with, then and only then, was he willing to bring the healing. And that is exactly what happened. That's not to say that I am now an expert on humility, sincerity, deeper faith and openness. However, these issues have become areas of focus and repentance for me. That's what God blesses. My back troubles came to an end--by faith being put into practice. It brought me to a new beginning--a new Genesis.

If you go and read the actual book of Genesis from chapter 30 to the last chapter, you will find many incredible parallels to our modern-day troubles by looking at the lives of Jacob and his sons... especially Joseph.

Jacob got swindled by his own father-in-law into working twice as long as agreed upon. Later he fears for his life against his brother Esau and is separated from his family. Jacob even wrestles with God and acquires an injury. Today it would be classified as a disability. I read that account many times before it registered with me that God gave him the disability. I therefore had to ask, "Did God give me my own disability?" Why would he do that?

Clues to that question are embedded in the book of Genesis. Much later, Jacob is lied to by most of his sons and falsely thinks his dear son Joseph has been killed. Imagine all the suffering this man went through. Yet did not God make him into a great nation? It was by faith that he endured these troubled times.

Genesis continues with the trials of Joseph. He is sold by his family and abandoned. He is falsely accused and left for dead in prison. Yet again, God delivers him, gives him a plan and the means to survive a severe famine, and makes his people into a prosperous nation.

How did Joseph endure through his bad times? Like his father Jacob, in his darkest despair, Joseph had to rely on the only one who could completely deliver him from slavery and dungeons. That is the God who saves. I am reminded of the scripture from 2 Corinthians 1:9 about why we sometimes fall into hard times:

"...this happened that we might not rely on ourselves but on God, who raises the dead."

Joseph in Egypt: an Attitude to Imitate

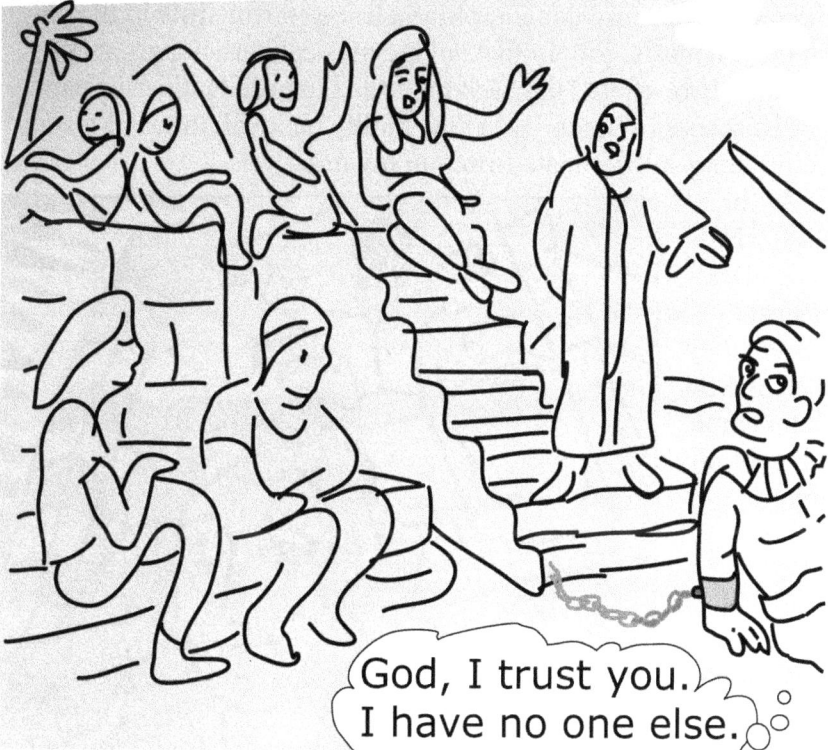

God, I trust you. I have no one else.

In good times and in bad, I believe Joseph was rewarded for his trust, as well as his consistent attitude of righteousness... no matter who was around or not around to see it. He did not give in to the sinister advances of Potiphar's wife. He had a commitment to purity, which is what we all need--that same heart. Without God, it is impossible to have and maintain such a heart. That is why daily prayer and Bible study with application will take our lives to the level that pleases God. This is the level that I hope and pray to meet all of my family and friends at, as fellow siblings in God's kingdom. It is the only level that will save us. It is the only level that will rescue the lost.

At the end of the musical *Joseph and the Amazing Technicolor Dreamcoat* (by Andrew Lloyd Webber and Tim Rice), there is an incredible climactic scene. Jacob and his presumed-dead son Joseph are reunited after years of separation. With all the triumphant drama that a musical can muster, the final round of lyrics starts with this song:

"So Jacob came to Egypt no longer feeling old and Joseph came to greet him in his chariot of gold... of gold!"

When I first saw this brilliant musical, I was more impressed with the fact that my daughter Maria had a starring role in the play and did a fantastic job. In fact, all the musical participants at her Riverside Brookfield High School turned in excellent performances.

The scenes of dreaming, envy, family betrayal, times of testing and rescuing still resonate firmly in my mind.

As for that final scene in the musical wherein they all sang, **"So Jacob came to Egypt no longer feeling old..."** I wondered why this was so climactic, aside from the concept that many theatrical productions end with a bang. I'm not completely dull. I do understand that father and son are finally reunited, so of course that's significant.

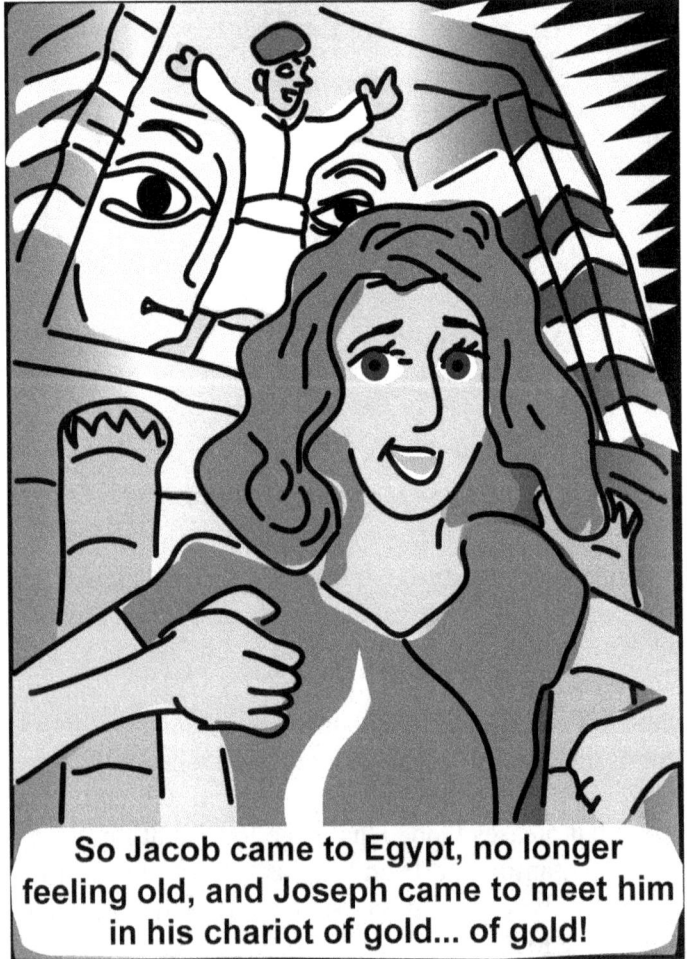

So Jacob came to Egypt, no longer feeling old, and Joseph came to meet him in his chariot of gold... of gold!

However, I felt as if I had missed a deeper issue. Perhaps I was distracted from the full meaning of the scene, because it was in this play that it fully hit me that my daughter was almost an adult. As she approached womanhood, I squirmed in my chair due to the back pain that made it unbearable to sit for more than a few minutes at a time. What else had I missed through the years squirming in pain? I may never know. Moreover, it had been at least a year since the last time I read through the book of Genesis.

Therefore, I went back and re-read the biblical version of the account of Jacob and Joseph in Genesis. Therein, I came to a profound understanding. The reason why this reunion is such a big deal is because of all the grief and hardships that father and son had been through--that God allowed them to go through. All those experiences, while super challenging, served to strengthen them as men in the faith. The unbearable trials didn't embitter these men. These trials softened their hearts, and God strengthened them.

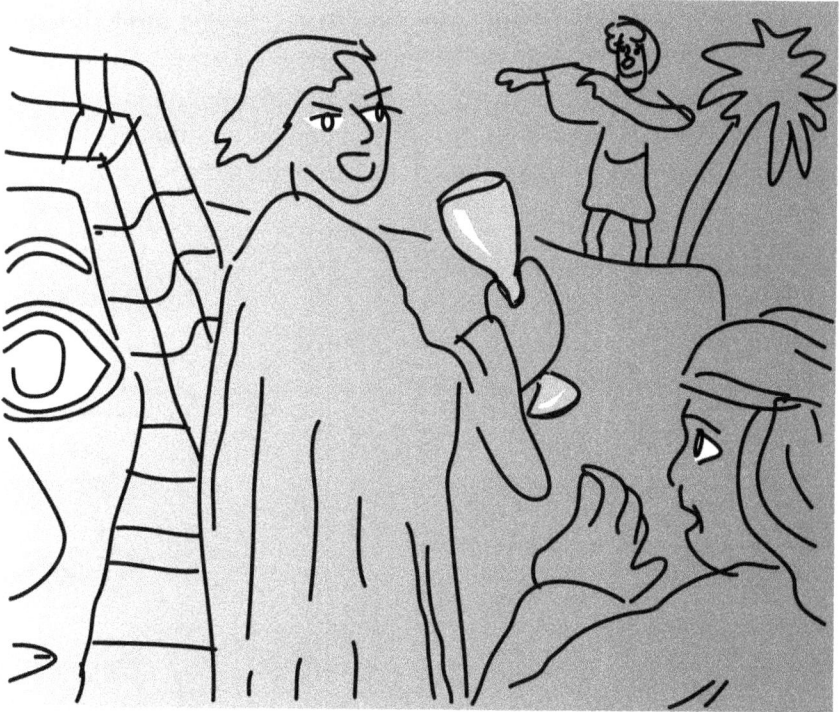

I believe that heroes like Jacob and Joseph had an anchoring faith about their final resting place. In the wonderful paradise of God, troubles and pains will be gone for good--no more need for them to be rescued or avenged. Their tattered and broken dreams, like the dazzling coat of Joseph, will be renewed in unimaginable ways, leaving them with the healing power of the Lord God Almighty.

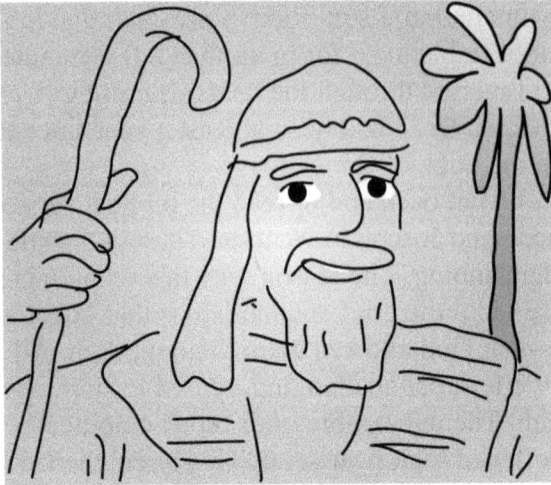

Just like Jacob and Joseph in the bygone centuries, God allows pains and troubles to happen to us today as well, to teach us what we need. He wants us to be survivors and point others into his rescuing hands. Moreover, if we do so, and if we keep putting matters in God's hands, won't we be clothed with the victor's crown and the dreamy colors of God in heaven?

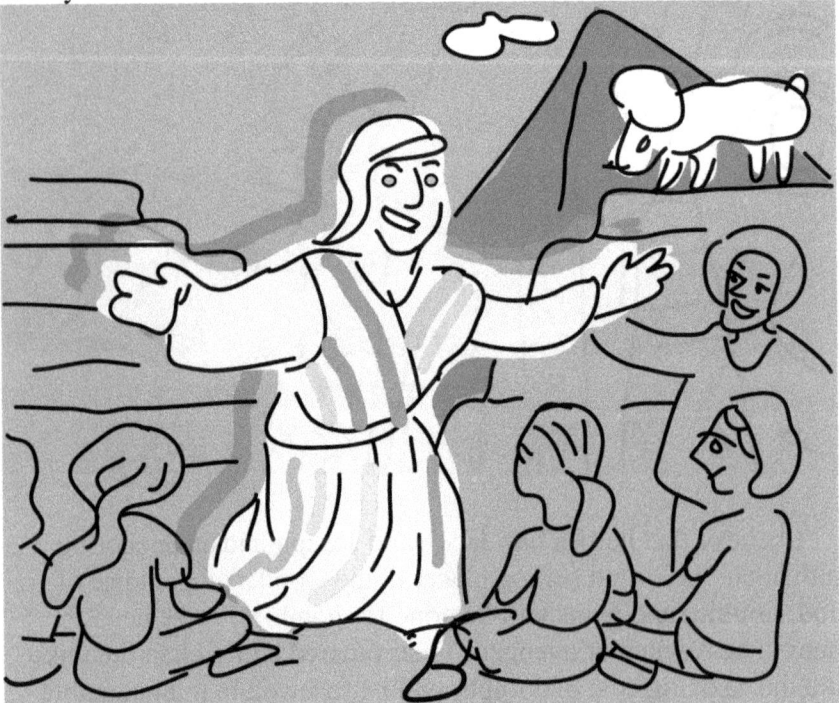

We will be like Jacob in eternity--no longer feeling old. We will be like Joseph in paradise--in a spiritual chariot of gold... of gold!

Chapter 14

Concussion Conclusions

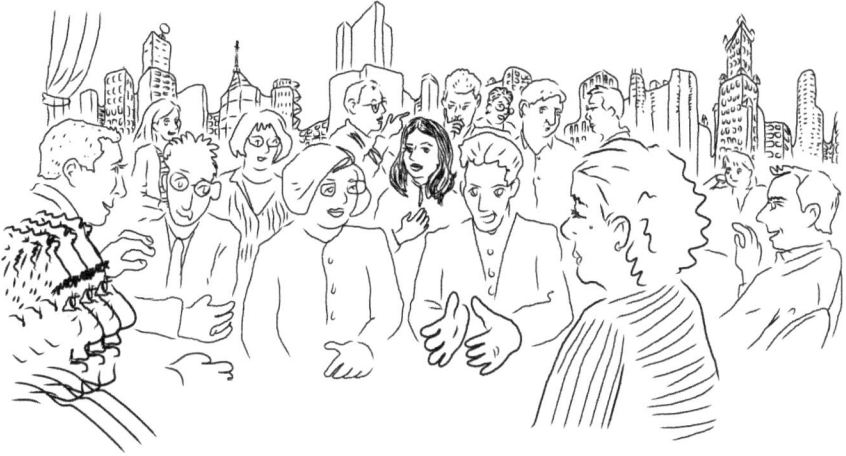

Today was a bigger-than-usual day for me. I met a former governor of Illinois, preached to the president and CEO of a massive business organization, and was told by my doctor to go to the emergency room because I probably have a concussion.

The concussion was from a car accident earlier in the week. I was the passenger in a stopped vehicle that got hit from behind by a big car going at least 20 miles per hour. Talk about back pain, this time the back of my head was the area of concern. My seat belt was on, so my head slammed forwards and then snapped backwards against the head rest, going so fast that nothing about it seemed to be restful. You know that feeling you get when stepping off of a speeding merry-go-round? That's how I still feel, and it's been four days since the crash.

Nevertheless, the prolonged dizziness did not stop me from attending and admiring a fine speech by former Governor "Big" Jim Thompson. He led the State of Illinois for 14 years, and the business leaders at the present-day event said that they missed him. Apparently, he did a better-than-average job as governor, since I can't recall anyone else in the business community speaking with such sincere public affection for any politician.

Indeed, Thompson's speech was quite excellent, calling us to think differently--on a multi-state level--and not just what's best for our own individual agendas. Moreover, it's hard not to enjoy any speech that quotes President Abraham Lincoln. Thompson reminded us of Lincoln's 1862 Civil War address to the US Congress:

"The dogmas of the quiet past are inadequate to the stormy present. The occasion is piled high with difficulty, and we must rise with the occasion. As our case is new, so we must think anew and act anew. We must disenthrall ourselves, and then we shall save our country."

After Thompson's speech, I had the pleasure of having a very nice chat with the top executive at one of Chicago's largest business associations. As we strolled down State Street, the conversation began with the usual for-profit business banter: high-level economic growth plans as well as how to understand what businesses need and how to help them tell their story.

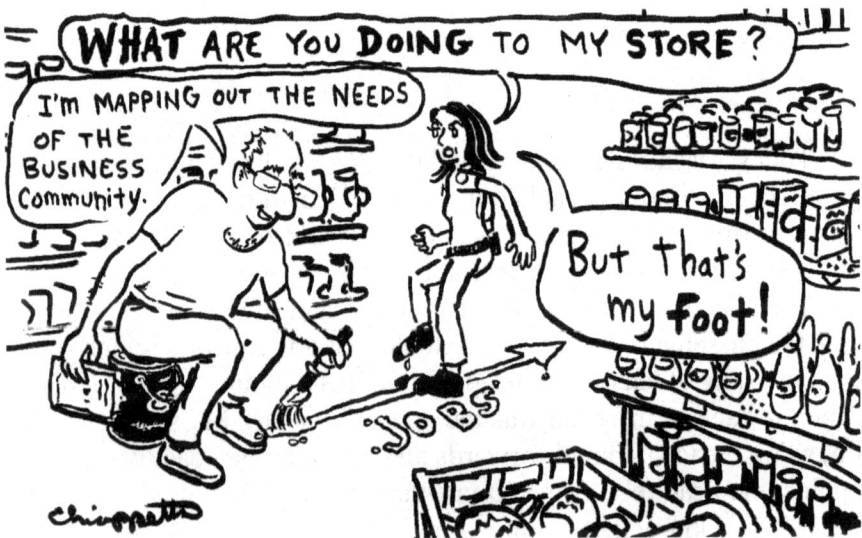

Such business talk is often interesting, yet never eternal. Therefore, I soon injected a spiritual element into our discussion. After a glance of endearment to the CEO, I told him something I had been hoping to bring up for months. "You would make a great disciple of Jesus Christ!" This man really is dear to me, yet his days are more obviously numbered with age and poor health.

"What does that even mean?" asked the CEO, who was somewhat religious, yet not committed to the lifestyle that Jesus calls us all to be fully engaged in.

I thought a moment before answering; "Just like I would come to you to learn and be your "disciple" if I wanted to learn about business, in much the same way, you need to come to a disciple of Jesus and learn from that disciple about how to follow Jesus. As you know, I am a disciple of Jesus and would be honored to show you the path that God has marked out for those who love him and desire to do his will."

Intrigued, the CEO asked, "So what would you teach me?"

I replied and sent up a quick prayer for God to open his heart, "I would teach you to seek first God's kingdom."

"How does a person just go and do that?" was the CEO's follow-up question.

I explained, "Jesus has an economic development plan that will blow your mind. His vision for the world is that everyone gets a chance to hear the good news about what he did for us."

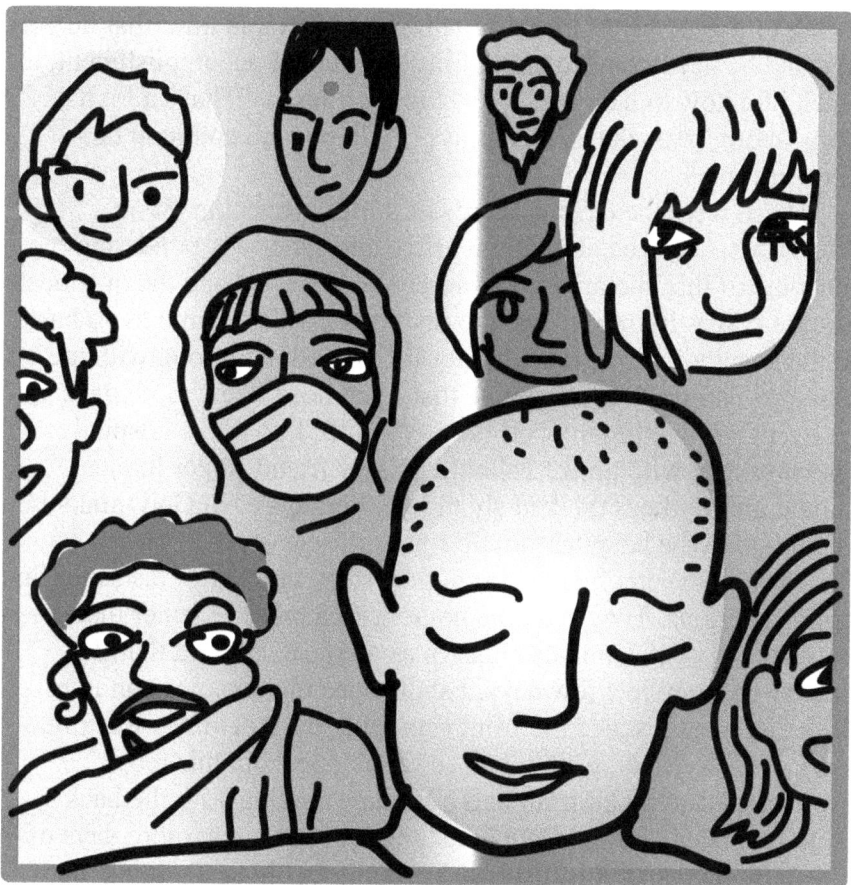

There were no objections or attempts to change the subject, so I continued; "It's about storing up treasure, not on earth, but in heaven.

Unless you make this the priority in your life, though, you will never fully understand what I am talking about. It's like trying to explain economic development to me if I was merely a random tourist with barely five minutes to soak up a few fun facts. We both know that would never work. In the same way, God's kingdom is his priority. The souls that will be with God in paradise are those who make God's kingdom a priority in their own lives now. This is what you need to do. It's what we all need to do."

As directly as I could, I concluded, "I am calling you to let me show you how to seek first God's kingdom. Make his plan your plan. Let's sit down, study the Bible, and live it out before the curtain closes on your life, or mine."

At this point in our walk, we came to the place where he had to break off to go to his office. As we parted, it was clear that he was trying to digest the mouthful of what I had just told him: that he was lost and he needed me, a man of little esteem or accomplishment, to teach him how to have a relationship with Jesus. "That's a lot to think about," was the CEO's reply. "We'll have to continue this another time."

Those were the closing words of our conversation. Soon afterwards, I arrived at my own office and sat down, pondering the outcome of this encounter. My adrenaline receded and the dizziness returned. Was it time to listen to my doctor? Was it time to go back to the hospital? I imagine that they'll find nothing wrong with me that they can fix. I also imagine that I just need a few more days to recover from getting my bell rung. Yet still, I go to the hospital anyways. My wife thinks I should go. My friend Roger thinks I should go. My boss thinks I should go. Perhaps even God thinks I should go to the hospital too. So I go.

Once in the emergency room, they run a number of tests and find nothing serious. They send me home with a piece of paper that says I have a head contusion, also known as a bruise. I'm told that if it doesn't go away in a few days, I should see my doctor. I can live with that. God rescued me from agonizing back pain. He was my Back Pain Avenger. Surely he can rescue me from this too.

I learned so much from half a lifetime dealing with the back pain. I wonder what he wants me to learn from a few more days of dizziness. Perhaps, it is just as Abraham Lincoln said: "think anew, and act anew." Perhaps in turn, Honest Abe was merely paraphrasing the words of the Apostle Paul from Romans 12:2:

"Do not conform to the pattern of this world, but be transformed by the renewing of your mind."

Whatever the case, both phrases are words to live by. As the world spins around the sun, and as the room spins around in my mind, I will ponder the mighty deeds of the Back Pain Avenger. He didn't just heal me; he made me better. I pray also in this case of dizziness, that he not only heals me, but also that he renews my mind to be more like his. Such a task would be insurmountable for one lone man such as me. Yet I choose to be one who thinks anew and acts anew. I choose to be in the mighty hands of the Back Pain Avenger, where all things are possible.

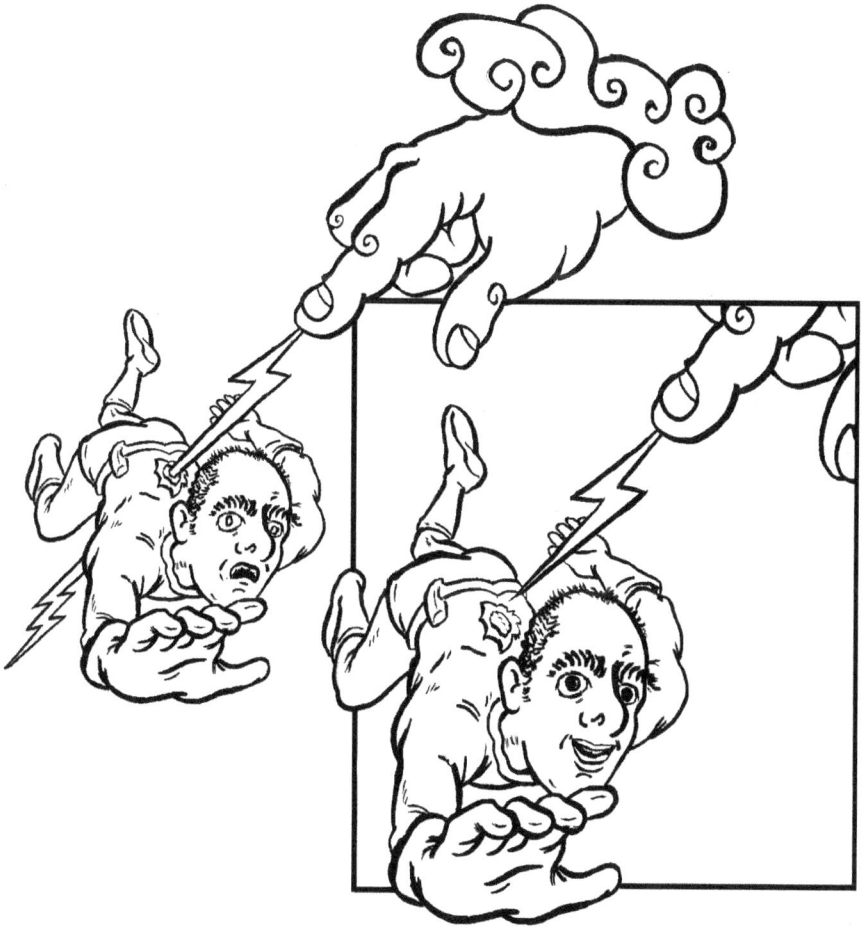

In Sickness and in Health

A Spouse's Perspective by Denise Chiappetta

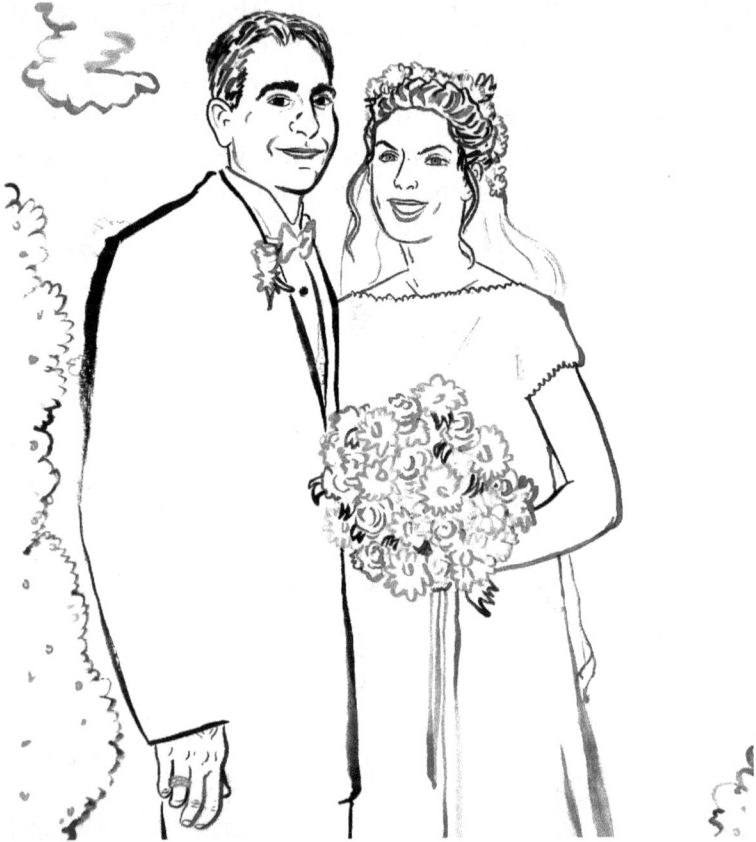

I've heard it said that healthy communication is a foundation for a great marriage. Perhaps. However, though my husband Joe and I now have a great marriage, our communication was not always very healthy. In fact, several things about our life were not healthy for an extended period--his back was one of them.

There were days when the communication might go something like this:

Denise: "Can you go pick up the baby out of her crib and bring her here?"

Joe: "No, not really. I don't think I can."

Denise: "The trash needs to go out."

Joe: [Silence]

Denise: "I guess I should go shovel the foot of snow out there."

Joe: "I wish I could help, but that's just not something I can do anymore."

Joe: "What time will dinner be ready?"

Denise: "No idea. Maybe never. How about making yourself a sandwich? Go ahead and make me one too."

Matters weren't helped by the fact that much of this dialogue took place with me towering over him, him sprawled lying on his back on the kitchen floor in front of his computer, pillows propping up his head and the keyboard. Or, worse yet, with him literally hanging upside down from an inversion table in our bedroom. Upside down. The symbolism was too ironic to be funny. Lots of things seemed to have flipped upside down since that walk down the aisle a few years prior.

On our wedding day, my husband was the picture of life and good health. Handsome, tanned, radiant, strong. Then again, why shouldn't he be? He was marrying me, his adoring and youthful bride. In a land of people surrounded by seas of tragic romances, we had the good fortune to find each other. This was the good life and we were both happy to sign up for it.

As years passed, and his chronic back pain worsened, the "good life" had to make a few "reasonable accommodations" of its own. Vacation travel, car trips lasting more than twenty minutes and leisurely dining out while seated in a restaurant were all but non-existent. For my husband, sitting brought on excruciating pain. Was I really going to insist on torturing him with a romantic, candlelit five-course meal? Clever conversation while in pain is quite an arduous task. So, I learned to love doing things like eating a burrito while taking a walking tour. Well, I didn't always love it. Sometimes I would want to choke on the reality of being barely thirty years old myself, and feeling like I was married to an "old man."

Though the worst episodes of his back pain are not my fondest memories of our thirteen-year marriage, it proved to be a very productive time. I was forced to learn some things about my marriage and character that may have gone otherwise unrecognized.

First, I had to examine the origins of my security as a woman. Was I secure in my identity and sex appeal only when on the arm of my tough "Italian Stallion" of a husband? Thankfully, Joe had never been in a position of having to physically defend me in public, but did part of me enjoy knowing that he could--if he needed to--take down someone who might be a threat? The answer was "yes." For all the Gloria Steinem books I read while in my teens and twenties, that damsel in distress/knight in shining armor scene still held some appeal. So would my devotion remain if my knight was sidelined and couldn't get up on horseback anymore?

In his *Back Pain Avenger* narrative, Joe confessed to not wanting to be identified as a person with a disability for a time. Well, I didn't really want to be identified as the wife of one either. It didn't fit with the description I pictured signing up for on that dotted line of marriage. Sure, I said, "In sickness and in health" on our wedding day. But, even though the word "sickness" technically preceded "health," it was easy to miss, especially with such a strong and radiant man in front of me at the time.

I had to face not only the chinks in the armor of my own self-esteem, but also fear in general. What if he never got better? What if he got worse? What if we never went on vacation or out to eat ever again? What did it really take to keep me happy? What if he lost his job and was permanently incapacitated? What if I had to become the breadwinner of the family? What if we lost our health insurance? What if he couldn't play ball or run with our kids? What if this chronic pain changed his very being and personality? What if he ceased to be the man I fell in love with? At the end of that litany, one thing seemed obvious: I needed a Back Pain Avenger as much as he did! While his back pain could physically stop him in his tracks some days, my fears could emotionally and spiritually do the same to me. Oh, come quickly Back Pain Avenger! We both need rescuing!

The Old Testament book of Isaiah 35:3-6 sheds some remarkable light on the situation:

"Strengthen the feeble hands, steady the knees that give way; say to those with fearful hearts, 'Be strong, do not fear; your God will come, he will come with vengeance; with divine retribution he will come to save you.' Then will the eyes of the blind be opened and the ears of the deaf unstopped. Then will the lame leap like a deer, and the mute tongue shout for joy. Water will gush forth in the wilderness and streams in the desert."

It is notable that this passage not only talks of God's power healing people with disabilities, but also addresses "those with fearful hearts." Okay, so he had a disability. I had a fearful heart. Both felt like a wilderness crying out for "streams in the desert." In both instances, it is God who rescues.

I was forced to examine the origins of my faith. Was Jesus truly the "author and perfecter" of my faith as he is referred to in the New

Testament book of Hebrews (12:2)? Did my faith thrive only when my circumstances were favorable and life was going the way I wanted it to? Is such a "faith" even truly faith? Scripture defines faith as **"being sure of what we hope for, and certain of what we do not see."** (Hebrews 11:1) Did my hopes for protection and security come from my husband's ability to live up to the duties I expected of him as a husband, or did my hope and security come from a deep trust in God? If all evidence of worldly security faded, did I still have hope, for myself, my husband, or life in general? If I truly believed God was my Lord and Savior, did he not deserve my trust and love in good times and bad? As Job asked his wife when hard times fell upon them, **"Shall we accept good from God, and not trouble?"** (Job 2:10)

I had to reckon with, not only the shallow conditions I put on my relationship with God, but my tendencies toward conditionals in my love for my husband. 1 Corinthians 13:4-8 has a lot to say about love and the bar is set high, based off of God's perfect love for his creation:

"Love is patient, love is kind. It does not envy, it does not boast, it is not proud. It is not rude, it is not self-seeking, it is not easily angered, it keeps no record of wrongs. Love does not delight in evil but rejoices with the truth. It always protects, always trusts, always hopes, always perseveres. Love never fails."

What a high calling, even during the "honeymoon" phase of a marriage! So what about in the hard times? The singer John Mellencamp popularized a song called "Jack and Diane." Some lyrics of note are: **"Oh yeah, life goes on, long after the thrill of living is gone... Hold onto sixteen as long as you can. Changes come around real soon, make us women and men."** Simply put, it was time for my commitment to love and my marriage vows to grow up. This wasn't a sixteen-year-old summer romance, this was my husband, my marriage, and both were worth fighting for, as well as sacrificing for.

I found that even in the hardest of days during his back pain, there was always something to be grateful for and a reason to "stay in love" with my husband. While he may not have been able to shovel the snow, or carry the baby around in her carrier as I may have wished, I could not deny his deep love and care for me and our children. Had he not been a man who continually prayed to God for strength, many of my aforementioned fears may have become reality. However, watching him leave for work, knowing what pain lay ahead of him for the rest of his day, traveling on a bus and train, holed up in an office, trying to concentrate while in constant discomfort, I had to admire his perseverance and commitment to provide for our family. Seeing him have courage in his weakness and then have the courage to face many of his own fears on an emotional level (not the most comfortable thing for a former "tough guy") I couldn't help but see a new type of strength in him and feel a renewed deep admiration. No, he wasn't the man I first fell in love with. He had been refined. He was better.

Looking back, we both became better. And I am faithful that we will continue to have much to look forward to, whether we are standing, sitting, or lying side by side.

Denise Chiappetta, 2012

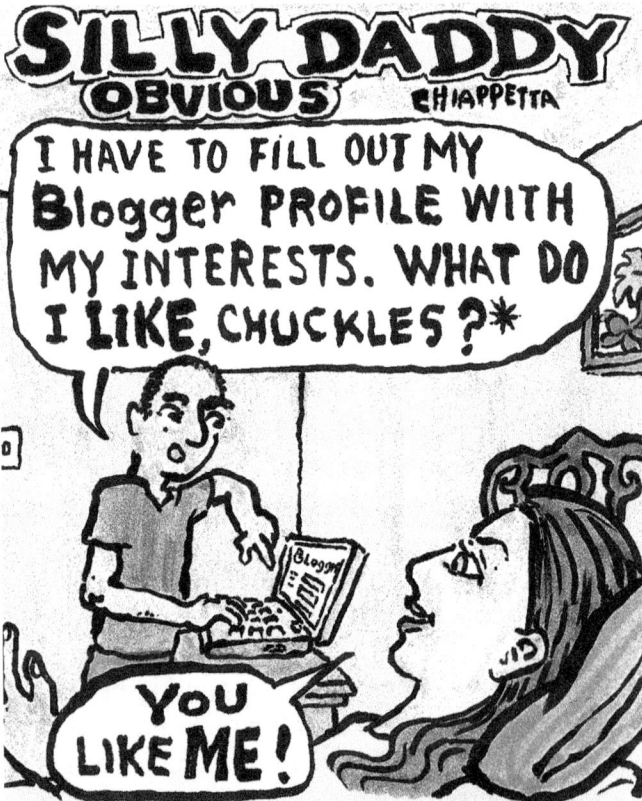

My Imaginary Friend

By Jillian Moyet

*An Abridged History of Having
Generalized Anxiety Disorder*

For almost as long as I can remember, I've not been in the world alone: I always had someone with me. Initially a stranger, we grew inseparable as time went on. It was his job, he said, to take care of me.

This friend of mine knew everything. He told me that great, ship-sized Man O' War jellyfish patrolled the oceans, that a sea monster lived in my drain, and that a bent and terrible figure was lurking out of sight; more normal jellyfish still managed to find their way into my bathtub, poised to sting me, and deadly bacteria grew everywhere.

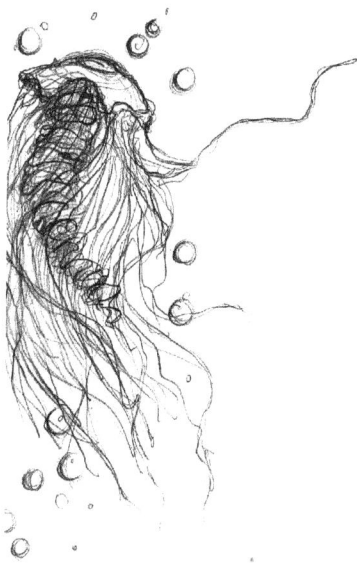

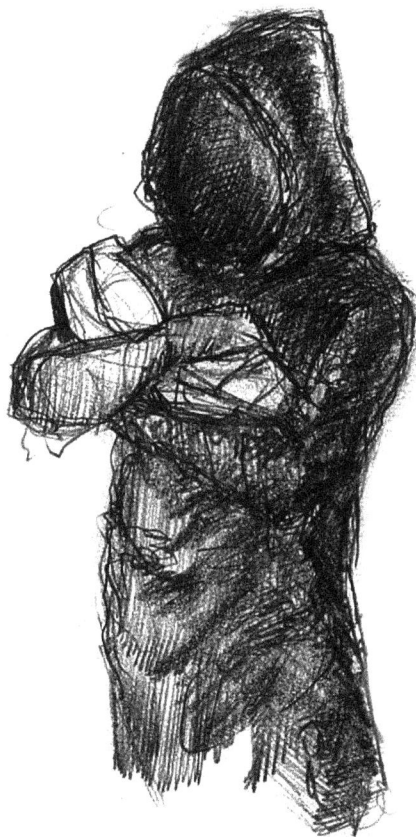

I navigated the world like a soldier in a minefield. Danger was never far away, and my friend was savvy enough to spot it for me. He was always telling me where to step (nowhere), what to avoid touching (everything), when to wash my hands (continuously), and what terminal illnesses I had contracted (it depended on the day).

There came a day when he insisted that we spend no time apart; I couldn't have a moment to myself alone. He was always at my side, distracting me from my schoolwork, my reading, my artwork, my family, and my

123

ability to think beyond whatever he said. He overwhelmed me, and I couldn't take it, even if it was for my own good, like he told me it was.

He constantly dictated my actions and doled out rules for survival, judging every misstep and calculating every mistake like a maniacal Pharisee. Do this, don't do that. Do you want to die? Listen to me or you will. Nothing I did was good enough or safe enough and I obsessed over the minutiae of my life and my thoughts. He hounded me day and night, always with new advice, and never letting me alone beyond a few brief moments. Life became a never-ending mantra of tasks and apologies. The day came when I would get in the car and almost wish for an accident, just to shut him up once and for all.

I had never been strong, but I pancaked under the enormous weight of his personality. In my distress I could think of only one person who could possibly have any control over this situation. I called out to him from where I lay curled up like a child and screamed at him, "This is your fault! You did this to me!" I was angry, and willing to blame God for all of my anguish and suffering. Why had he put me in such callous hands? How did he expect me to stand up against it all?

On my own, I could not feel. My thoughts were dead and I couldn't identify my own emotions. Sometimes I felt like a pair of eyes looking out at the world.

I grew reckless and apathetic. I would bankrupt myself to derive what pleasure I could out of life. I would spend my

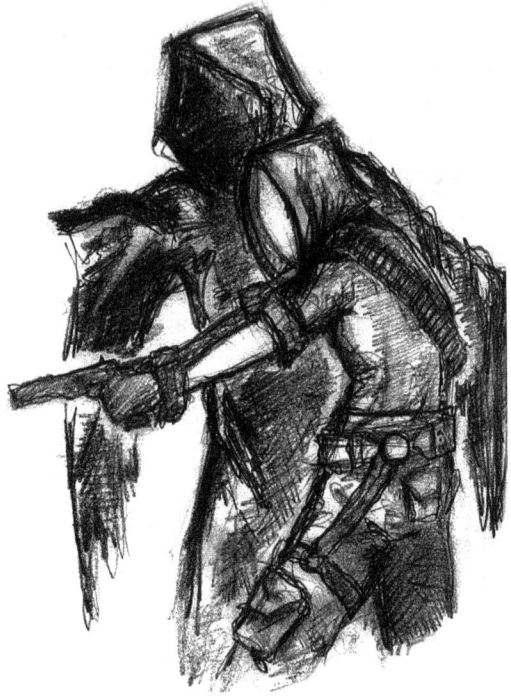

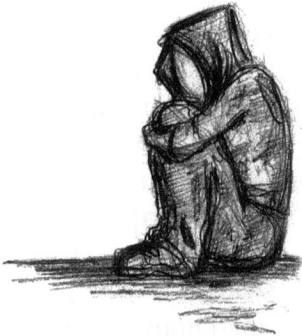

money rashly and put myself into debt with banks almost regularly. I consumed food like a glutton, when I bothered to eat at all. The things I did to distract myself from him never worked for long; they only made my situation worse, and gave him a stronger foothold.

He drove me crazy. Because of him I suffered panic attacks, depression, exhaustion, paranoia, and pains that I could never account for. My back and my limbs would ache, my extremities would tingle, and my sleep was irregular. I saw things that weren't necessarily real. My vision had short-circuited and my brain saw the strangest things in the most mundane scenery.

Eventually, I was told to get medication, and when I did, he seemed to fade away, though not without a fight, and never out of my sight from where he occasionally stalked the corners of my vision. But he was, for the most part, gone.

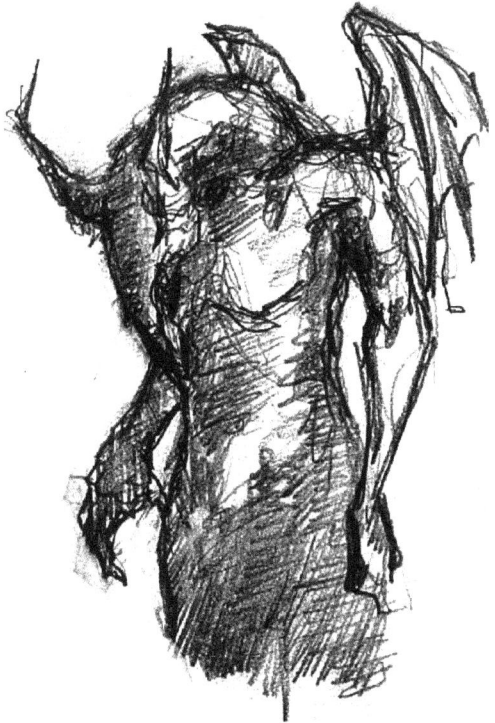

Years later, I lay in bed one lonely night, terrified. He stood beside me, very close to me again, and more concerned for my welfare than usual. I had been prescribed some new medication and it was having some good effects on me, but he tried to convince me to stop taking it.

"That was no normal stomach ache you had not long ago," he told me, "even if the hospital gave you an explanation. And that nausea you felt tonight? It's got to be a side effect and a bad one. And now you're suffering this horrible panic attack for some reason! If you keep taking this medicine, I promise you that you'll die." I felt so terrible that I felt he could be right.

Again I thought about the one person who had control over all of my life, and everything my friend said seemed to make sense. It felt like God had planned all this. It felt like I was going to die.

"He's not pleased with you," my friend said. "You're a lost cause to him. He's going to remove you completely if you let him. But I can help you."

I wanted so much to never take my medicine again. I wanted so much to give in to his protection like I always did, even if I'd grown to hate him and had been happy without him. Yet, as I struggled through the night, it occurred to me that this all might be a lie. The more I thought about it, the less sense his assertions made.

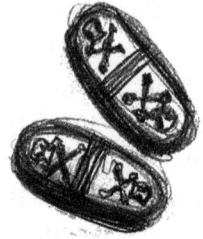

"Why would God do that to me?" I asked.

And for once, my friend had no answer!

As morning came, all I could do was call out to God to help me. And all the time my friend stood at my side, practically begging with me to not do what I was about to do.

I eventually did rise from bed, and I felt pulled in two from both sides, but I didn't stop until I'd swallowed my morning dosage, and by then there was no turning back. I reasoned that, either way, I'd made my decision. I started to see a better way: that God was not trying to sabotage me. God wasn't going to push me away.

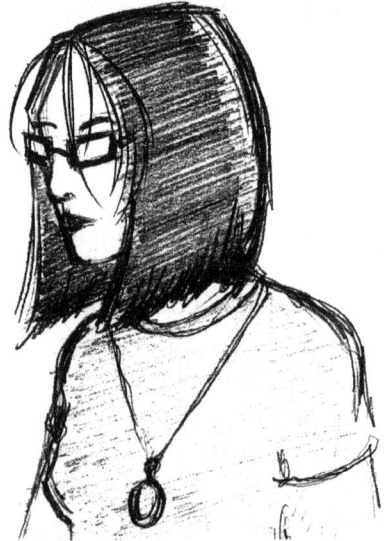

The stranger from my youth is not as loud now, but he still waits for me to come back and return things to the way they used to be. He still follows me around, and still badgers me. He's there when I wake up and he's there when I go to sleep. He follows me on the train and sits with me at work.

But we're not friends anymore.

"'For I know the thoughts that I think toward you,' says the LORD, 'thoughts of peace and not of evil, to give you a future and a hope. Then you will call upon me and go and pray to me, and I will listen to you.'" (Jeremiah 29:11-12)

Jillian Moyet, 2012

Disability in Comics

A Celebration of Characters with Disabilities in the History of Comics Spanning One Thousand Years

Researched by Joe Chiappetta

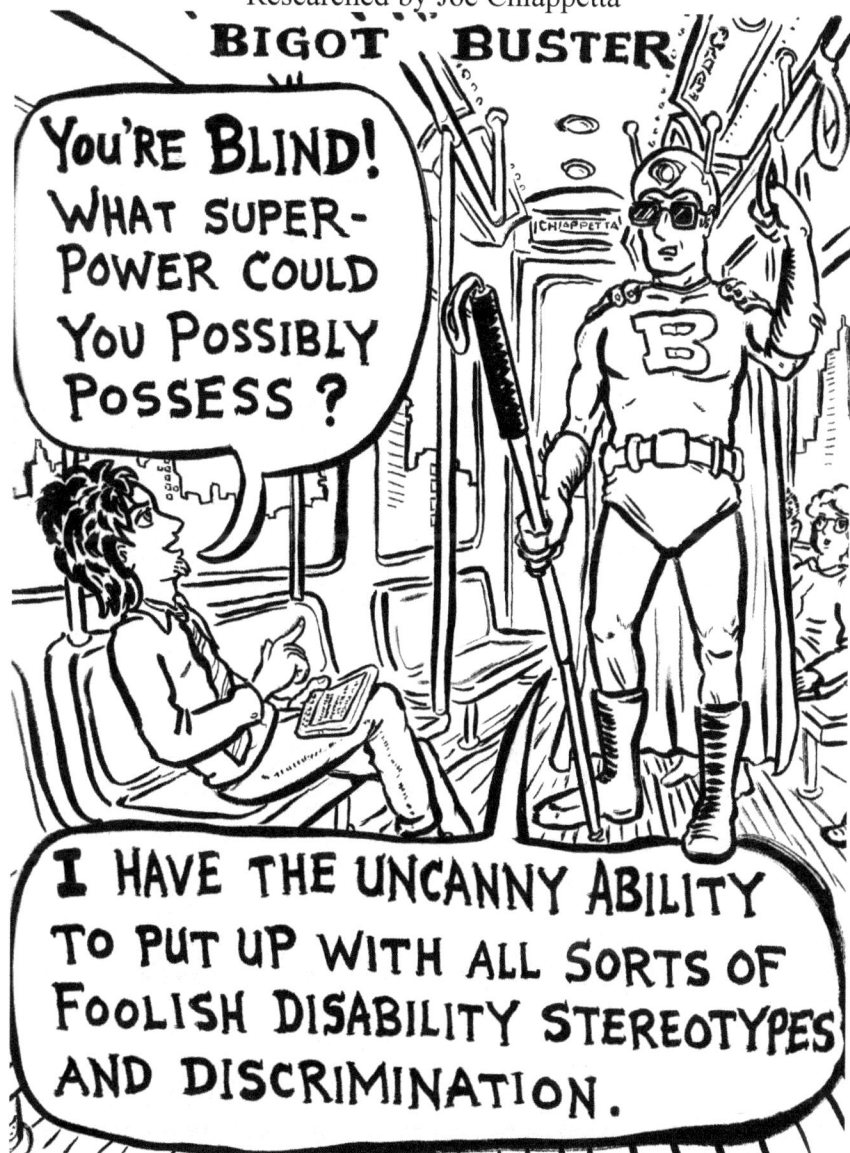

Clearly, the heroic work of the Bigot Buster is never done. Mention comic books or comic strips, and the last thing that comes to mind for most people would be disability issues. Yet a deeper look into the history of comics reveals a very close connection. In fact, the more you look for disability topics in comics, the more you find. In fact, disability coverage in comics seems to appear in every century which comics also appear.

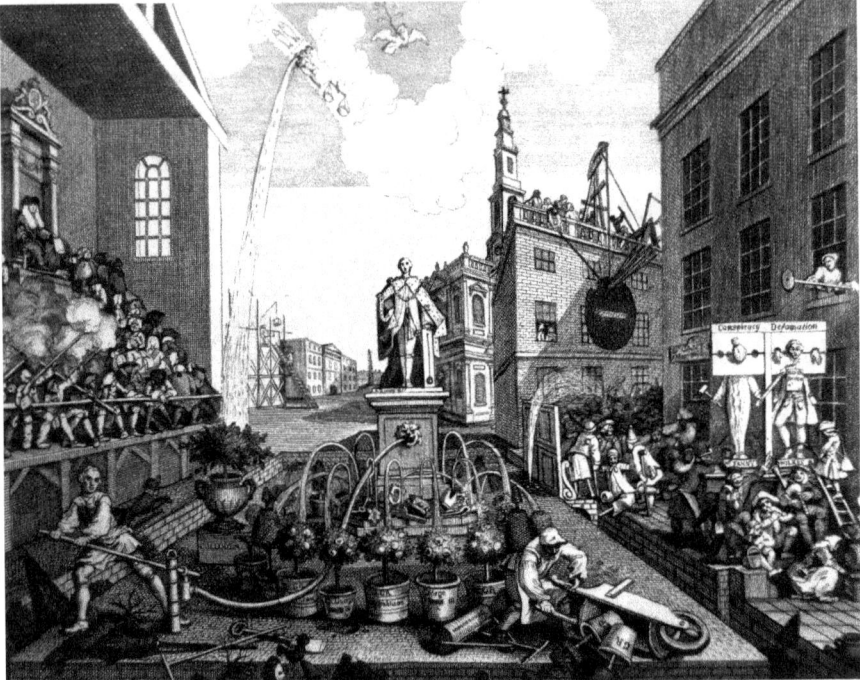

"The Times, Plate 2" by William Hogarth, 1762 (with detail below)

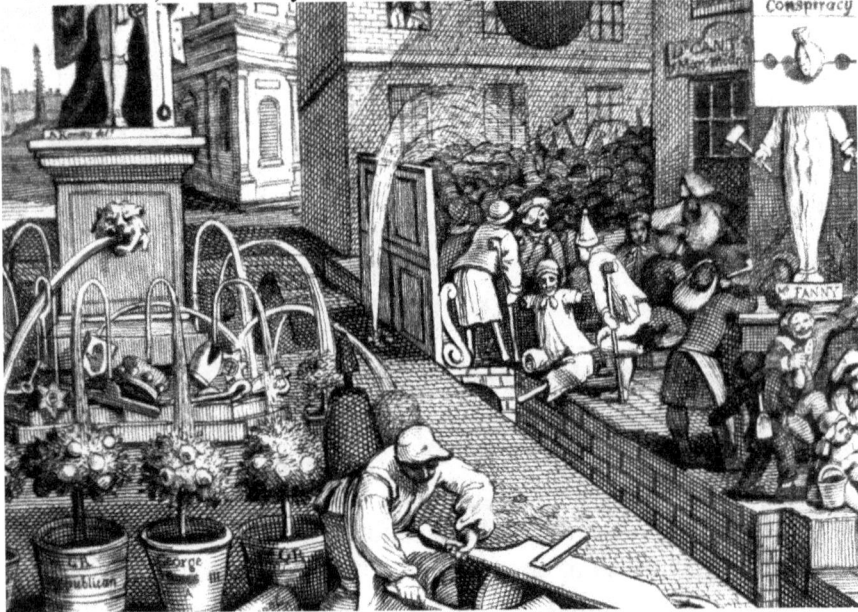

Near the end of his life, English artist William Hogarth drew an antiwar satire in 1762 called "The Times, Plate 2." Not only is it an early political cartoon, but it is also one of the earliest cartoons highlighting people with disabilities. Blocked from reaching King George III, who is represented by the statue at center, veterans with disabilities from the Seven Years War can be seen in the right portion of the cartoon with crutches as well as missing limbs.

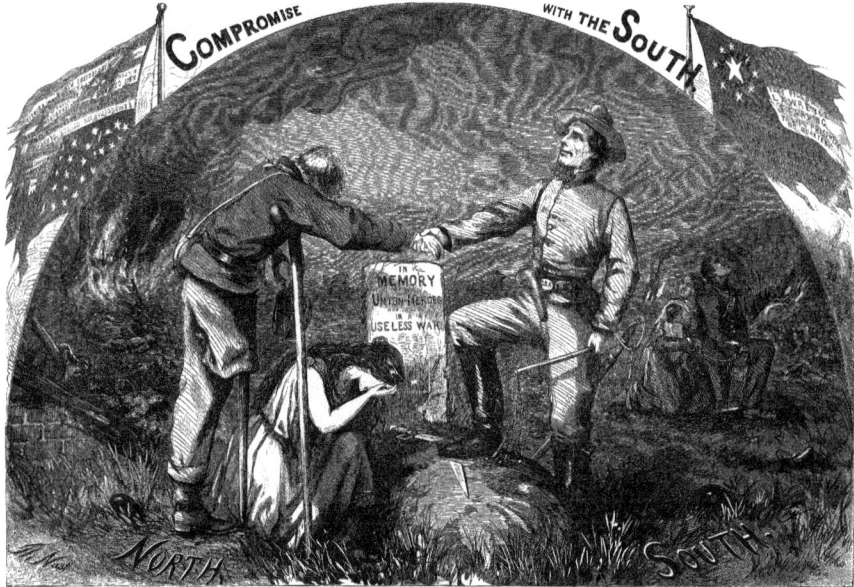

DEDICATED TO THE CHICAGO CONVENTION.

Thomas Nast's depiction of a Union soldier who has lost his leg in the Civil War served as an element in a powerful American political cartoon. First published in *Harper's Weekly* (September 3, 1864), viewers would think twice about an early compromise with the South after reading the charges on the Southern "slavery/treason" flag in the upper right corner. "Bayoneting the wounded" and "scalping" are some of the accusations written into the flag.

A closer look at the African-American family at right shows that they are again in chains. Nast made the case to Northern politicians looking to end the war prematurely that disabilities and deaths would all be in vain should the North back out before conquering the South.

Wounded warriors were a somewhat frequent theme in Thomas Nast's war

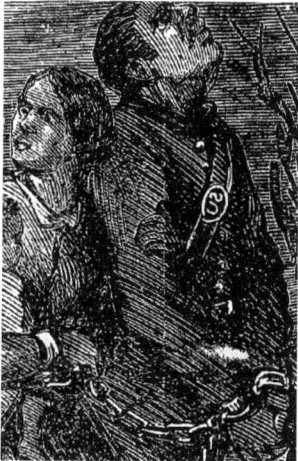

cartoons. Civil War soldiers with disabilities may even be the very first recurring characters with disabilities in American comics. Reproduced here in partial detail is Nast's seven-panel comic "Andrew Johnson's Reconstruction" (*Harper's Weekly* September 1, 1866). The complicated business of securing rights for African-Americans, while also healing a wounded nation is portrayed while a dishonorably discharged soldier with a disability stands watching as his arm lies severely bandaged from the elbow downward.

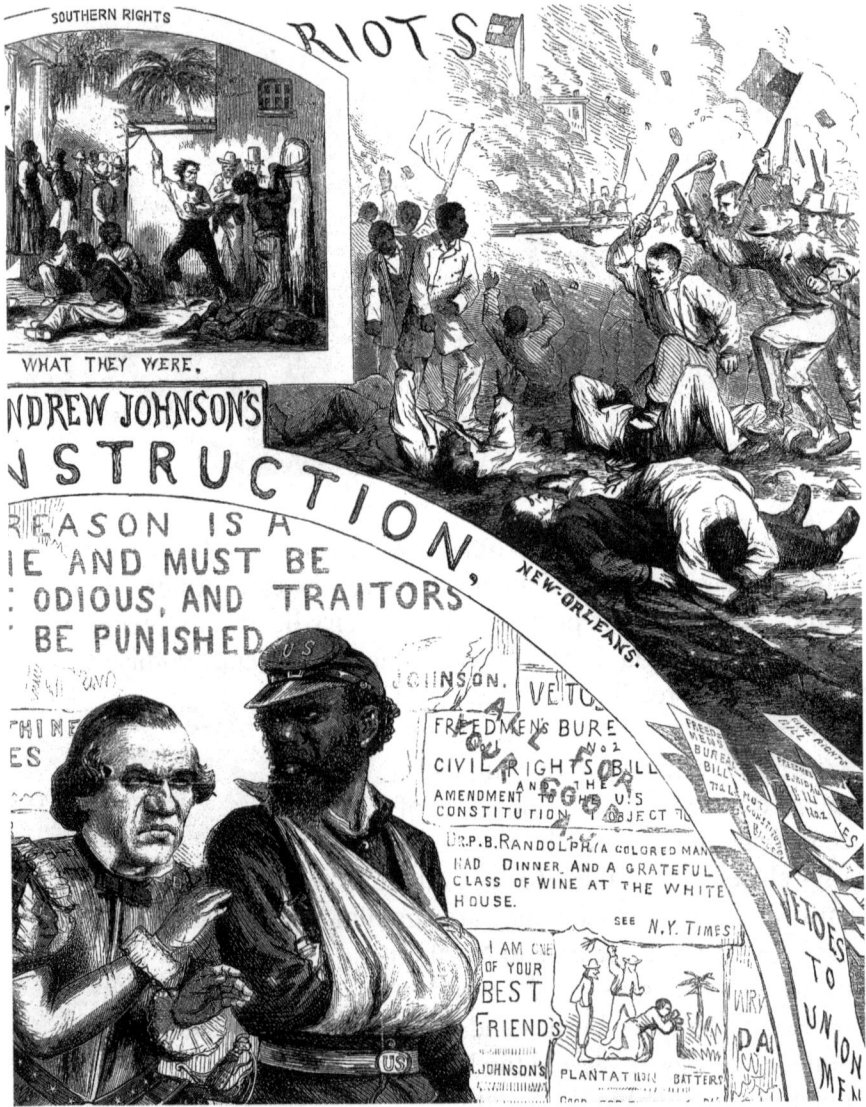

Only one fourth of "Andrew Johnson's Reconstruction" is reproduced here, to zoom in on the detail. Note the panels within panels, and the text-heavy integration with images. Not only is this cartoon an early depiction of disability in comics, but it is also one of the most innovative comics compositions, even by contemporary standards.

In 1874, Thomas Nast created the Republican Party's mascot, an elephant, which is still used today. By 1877, in *Harper's Weekly*, Nast gave that elephant multiple disabilities and a victor's crown to represent the hard-won presidential race and election of Rutherford Hayes.

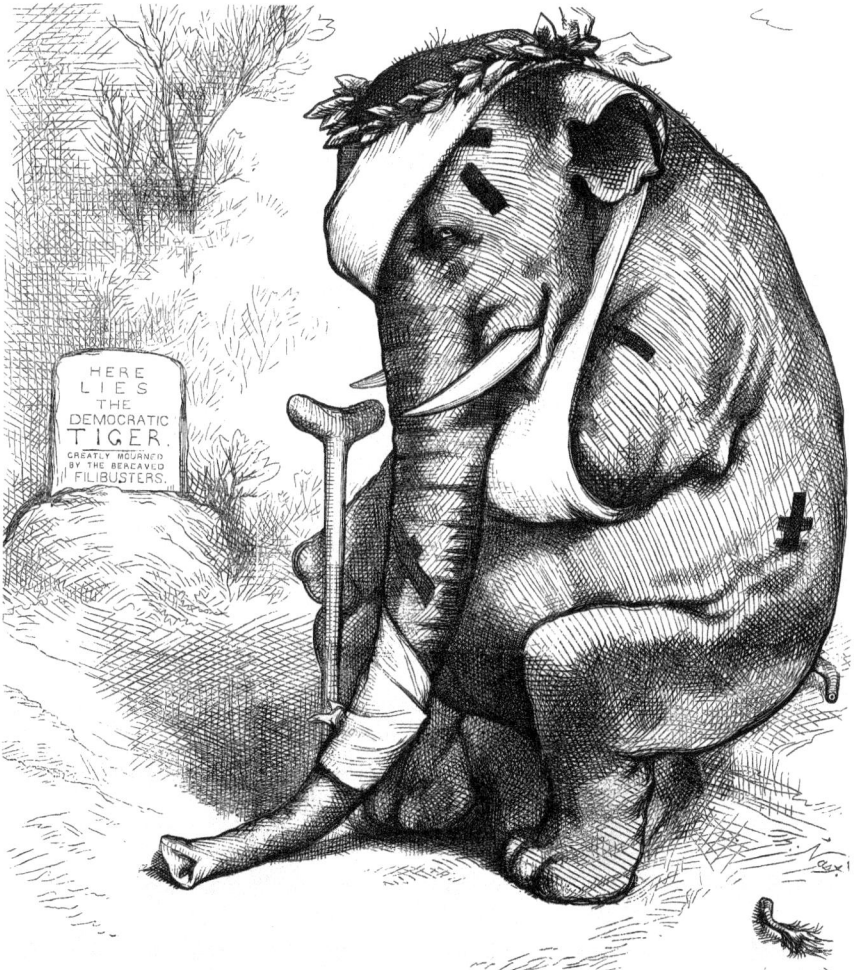

ANOTHER SUCH VICTORY, AND I AM UNDONE.--Pyrrhus

The elephant cartoon's caption is a quote from the ancient King Pyrrhus of Epirus, who defeated the Romans in 280 BC, but with a devastating amount of casualties.

Exploitation of disability appears in an 1892 cartoon by F.M. Hutchins. He created a three-panel comic for *Puck Magazine* called "The Fake Blind Man." Therein, a few shrewd kids match trickery with trickery and expose a pretender begging with dark glasses and a sign that reads "Please Help the Blind."

In 1896, Richard Outcault created a *Yellow Kid* cartoon for *New York World* called "Amateur Dime Museum in Hogan's Alley." The background of this comic depicts the grim realism of the times; a child accidentally gets shot in the eye when another youth sorely misses his mark at a shooting gallery booth. Without any commentary, the viewer can instantly take for granted that disability can happen to anyone at anytime.

The above works are only a small sampling from the history of comics wherein characters with disabilities are depicted in some fashion. While such a study is most fascinating, what follows is a non-exhaustive list of comics which *feature* disability issues or recurring characters with disabilities. Unlike the examples previously cited, priority will be given to comics that either have more than a brief brush with disability topics or comics that have leading characters with disabilities.

Moreover, since it is a widespread and damaging stereotype that most fictional villains have some sort of psychiatric impairment, more attention will be given to non-villains. Villains with mental illnesses will not be completely ignored, but priority will be given to characters--good or bad--who represent a wider range of disability categories.

From this list, it should be clear that the coverage of disabilities in comics has always been significant, but not always appropriate by today's standards of disability etiquette. What is encouraging is that instances of disability topics in comics do appear to be increasing as comics become a more accepted mode of cultural expression.

Note that inclusion of a specific work of comics into this list does not constitute a recommendation to read, or not to read these comics. Rather, for those interested in disability studies and comic history, it is important to see how commonplace disability issues in comics have been. Consider the following examples:

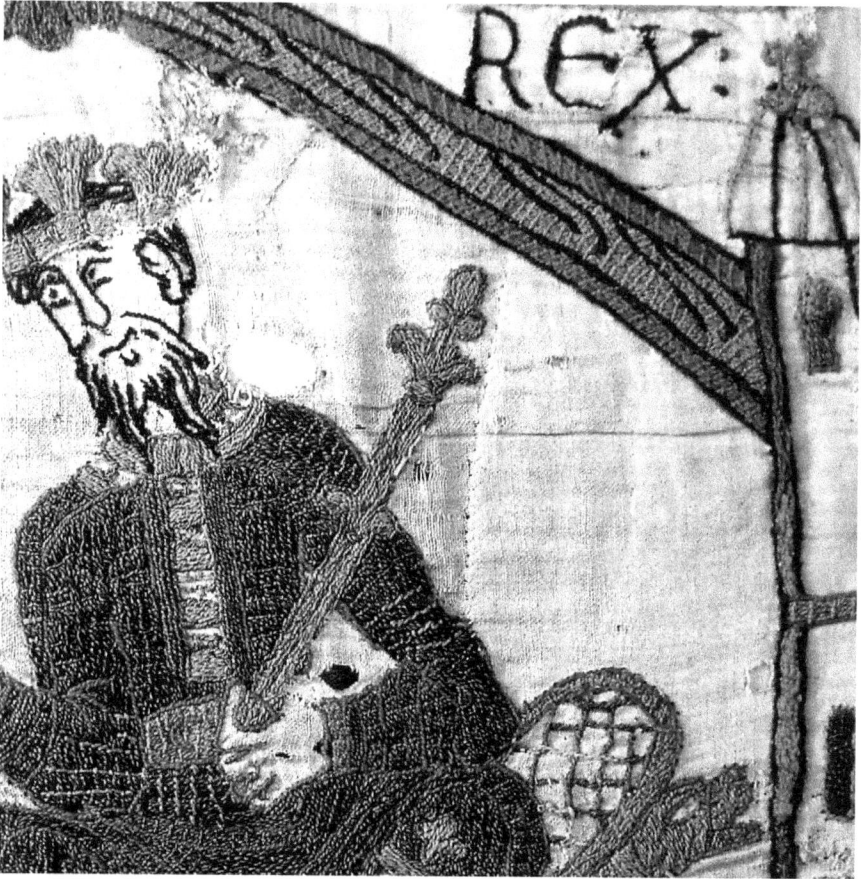

1070 AD: **King Edward with an undisclosed disability**. There is nothing quite like the Bayeux Tapestry in terms of identical surviving art forms from the Middle Ages, but perhaps its closest descendant would be the modern-day comic strip, or even graphic novel. King Edward was a real king and also one of the main characters in the Bayeux Tapestry.

Most intriguing for the study of disability in comics, this story of war between the English and the Normans also contains one of the earliest leading characters with disabilities in a comic format. King Edward of England, also known as Edward the Confessor, is shown at the beginning of the story holding a scepter on his thrown. At this point in the story he most likely does not have a disability.

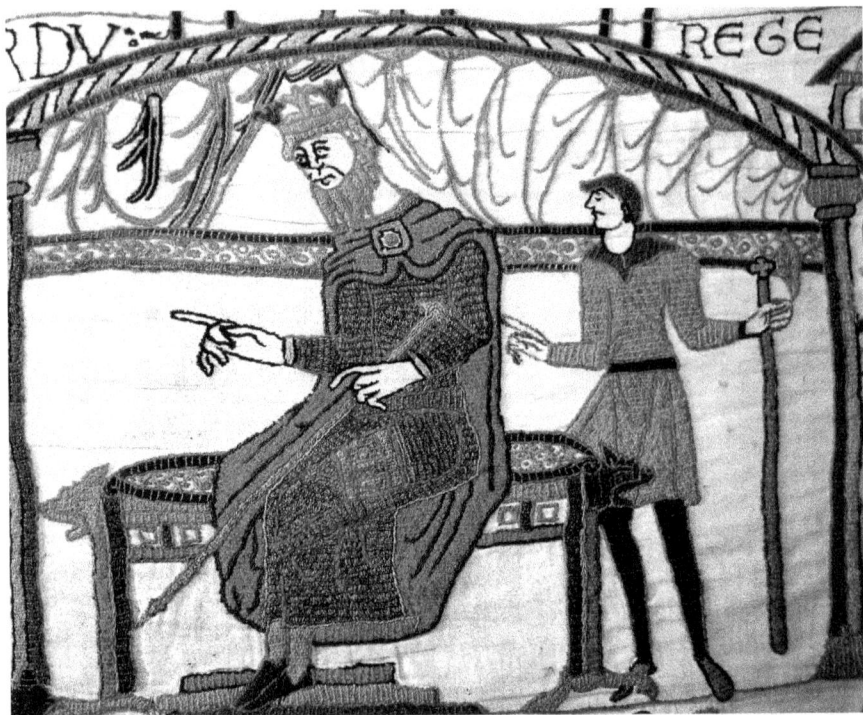

However, by the middle of the Tapestry, King Edward has replaced his ornate scepter for a plain walking stick. In the very next scene, his funeral procession is depicted, and then the story flashes back to just before his death. King Edward is shown on his sick bed, giving his final instructions to his loyal friends. Thus the ancient English King Edward goes down in history, not only as one of the most visually well-documented leaders of his era, but also as one of the first, if not the first, leading character with a disability in comics.

Created in 1070 AD in Europe, the Bayeux Tapestry is 230 feet long, and contains 50 sequential scenes with integrated captions describing the action. If this sounds like a comic, that's because it is a comic--a medieval one written in Latin to be precise.

According to historian Frank Barlow in "Edward the Confessor" (University of California Press, 1984), King Edward most likely had a number of strokes in the year before his death in 1066 AD. This may explain his use of a cane and his decline in health depicted toward the middle of the Bayeux Tapestry.

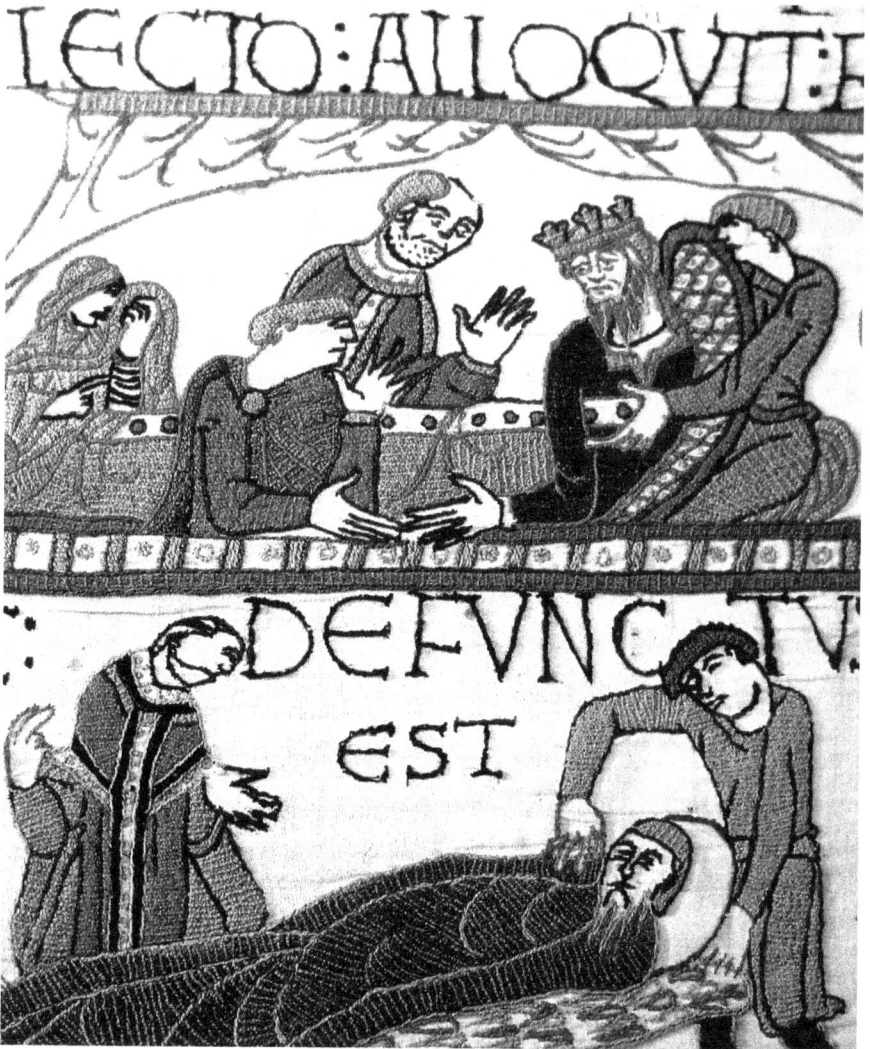

While not covered in the Tapestry, King Edward is also known as the king who defeated the Scottish King Macbeth. Though nearly 1000 years would pass before leading characters with disabilities might regain such prominence in comics, King Edward sets the bar high as a most impressive character with a disability.

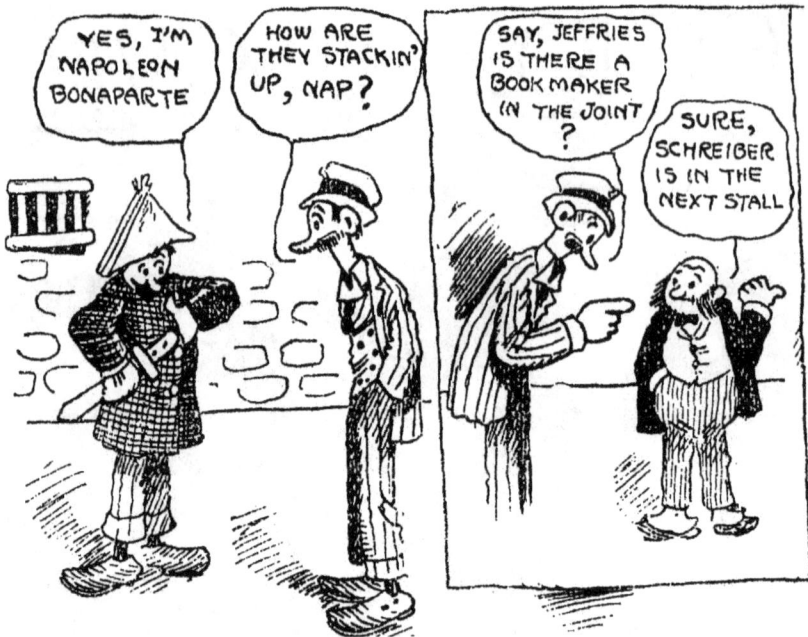

YES, I'M NAPOLEON BONAPARTE

HOW ARE THEY STACKIN' UP, NAP?

SAY, JEFFRIES IS THERE A BOOK MAKER IN THE JOINT?

SURE, SCHREIBER IS IN THE NEXT STALL

1908: **Jeff as a resident of a psychiatric institution** was created by Bud Fisher for the *Mutt and Jeff* comic strip. This series is considered the first daily newspaper comic strip. The first appearance of Jeff shows him as an inmate of a psychiatric institution where many are locked up for thinking they are famous people like Napoleon or champion boxers. Jeff eventually rejoins society to live a life of odd urban schemes with his new friend Mutt.

1929: **Popeye with a visual impairment** was created by E. C. Segar in the comic strip *Thimble Theatre*. Missing an eye, Popeye the sailor does not let that stop him from using his abilities for good. Later cartoonists have depicted Popeye with a squinty eye.

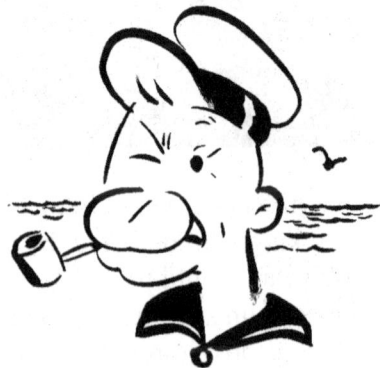

J. Chiappetta 2012
AFTER E.C. SEGAR 1929

1929: **Count Screwloose from Toulouse with a mental illness** was created by Milt Gross. Escaping from Nuttycrest, the count finds the outside world just as messed up and returns to the psychiatric institution. The comic strip was later adapted into a few animated cartoons by MGM.

136

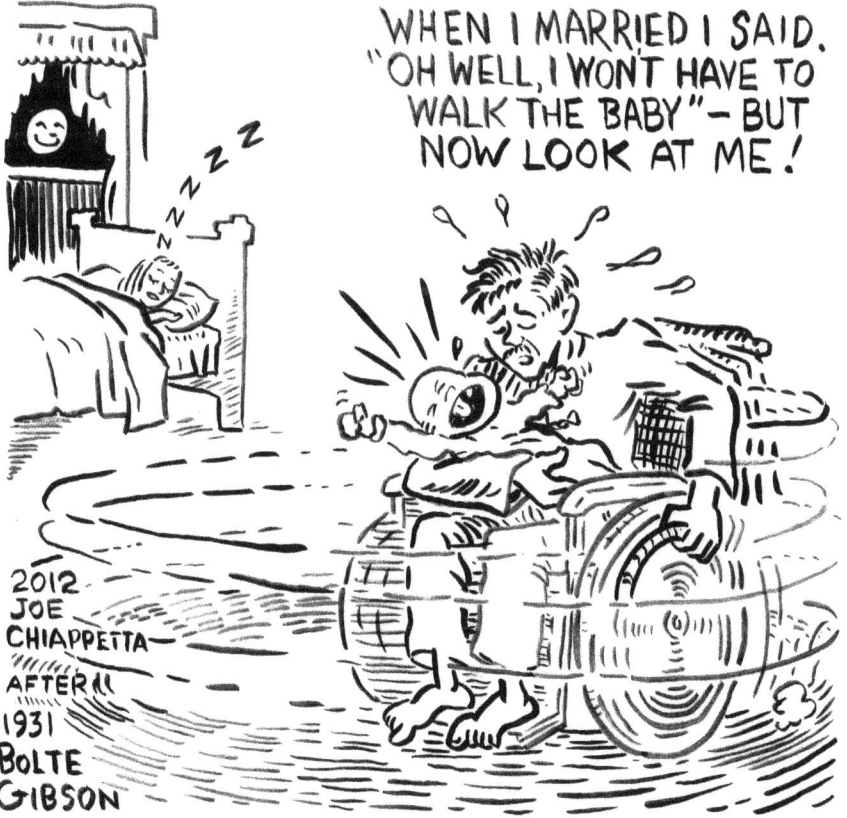

THE OLD PARAL SAYS –

WHEN I MARRIED I SAID, "OH WELL, I WON'T HAVE TO WALK THE BABY" – BUT NOW LOOK AT ME!

2012 JOE CHIAPPETTA AFTER 1931 BOLTE GIBSON

1931: **The Old Paral with poliomyelitis** was an otherwise nameless man with a mustache in the comic strip *The Old Paral Says* by Bolte Gibson for *The Polio Chronicle*. While the "Old Paral" appeared as more of a middle-aged man rather than as an old man, the comic strip featured a number of great insights into disability awareness themes, especially revolving around physical impairments.

The Polio Chronicle was published from 1931 to 1934 by the National Patients Committee at the Roosevelt Warm Springs Institute for Rehabilitation in Warm Springs, Georgia, USA. Franklin Delano Roosevelt was a founder of the Institute, and also a frequent visitor. Therefore it is very likely that the 32nd president of the United States of America was a reader of *The Polio Chronicle*. The Institute, while no longer publishing *The Polio Chronicle*, still serves people with disabilities today.

POLIO PETE

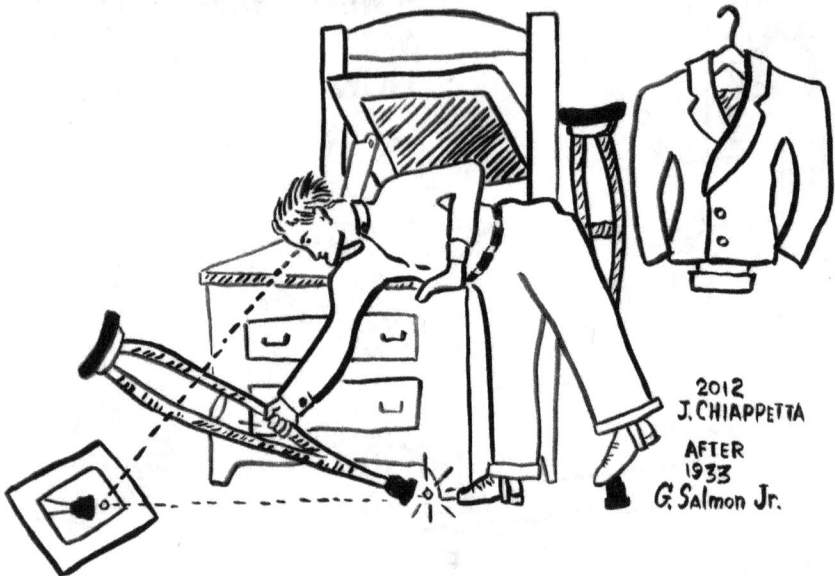

2012
J. CHIAPPETTA

AFTER
1933
G. Salmon Jr.

SEARCHING FOR THE MISSING LINK

1933: **Polio Pete with poliomyelitis** was created by G. Salmon, Jr. for *The Polio Chronicle*. Using his crutches, and at times a wheelchair, Polio Pete shows the adaptive nature of people with disabilities. Many of Pete's adaptation techniques are simply brilliant.

1940: **The Joker with a mental illness** was created by Jerry Robinson, Bill Finger, and Bob Kane of DC Comics (*Batman* #1). Having, perhaps, the most severe mental illness imaginable, The Joker, along with many super-villains, is a dangerously disturbed killer. In today's terminology, he might be diagnosed with antisocial personality disorder. He often ends up in Arkham Asylum, which is the psychiatric institution for many villains in the DC Universe.

1941: **Doctor Mid-Nite with blindness** was created by Charles Reizenstein and Stanley Josephs Aschmeier of DC Comics (*All-American Comics* #25). Blinded by a grenade, Charles McNider can mysteriously see in complete darkness to fight crime.

1941: **Captain Marvel, Jr. with mobility issues** was created by Ed Herron and Mac Raboy of Fawcett Comics (*Whiz Comics* #25). After losing the use of one of his legs to a super-villain, Freddy Freeman can walk (and fly) unassisted only in his superhero form as Captain Marvel, Jr. When not fighting crime, he reverts to using a crutch. He also uses a wheelchair at times.

1946: **Brilliant with blindness** was created by Chester Gould for the *Dick Tracy* comic strip. As inventor of the 2-Way Wrist Radio and many other Dick Tracy gadgets, Brilliant was a recurring minor character until he was killed off in 1948.

1948: As a **disability expert, Rex Morgan, M.D.** was the title of a comic strip and the main character created by Dr. Nicholas P. Dallis, a psychiatrist. Medical and disability issues were often central themes for Rex Morgan to tackle in his comic strip.

1949: **Moose Mason with a learning disability** was created in *Archie's Pal Jughead* #1 for Archie Comics. It was later specified that Moose has dyslexia.

1952: **Mister Magoo with a visual impairment** was a comic book character in *Gerald McBoing Boing and the Nearsighted Mr. Magoo*, published by Dell Comics. First appearing in animated

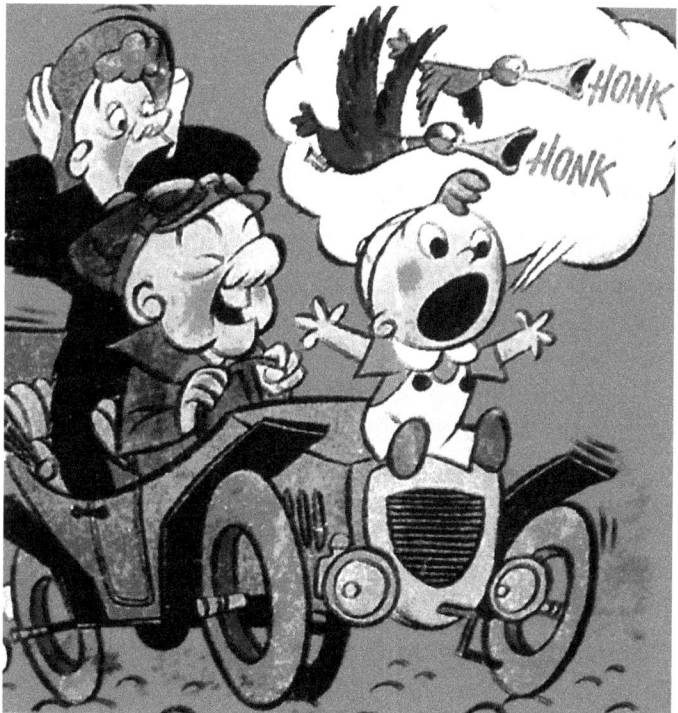

cartoons created in 1949 by Millard Kaufman and John Hubley of UPA, it remains questionable whether or not that Quincy Magoo's disability can be completely corrected with prescription glasses.

1962: **The Hulk with a mental illness** was created by Stan Lee and Jack Kirby of Marvel Comics (*The Incredible Hulk* #1). Having multiple personality disorder, Bruce Banner and his alter ego, the super strong, yet super simple Hulk, have saved the world on many occasions. The Hulk also has some sort of intellectual disability, but don't tell him that. He may smash you, puny human.

1962: **The Mighty Thor with mobility issues** was adapted from Norse mythology by Stan Lee, Larry Lieber, and Jack Kirby of Marvel Comics (*Journey into Mystery* #83). When Thor is in the human form of Dr. Donald Blake, he has a lame leg and walks with the use of a cane.

1963: **The Lizard with an amputation** was created by Stan Lee and Steve Ditko of Marvel Comics (*Amazing Spider-Man* (vol. 1) #6). When Dr. Curt Connors wounded his right arm, it was amputated. He created a serum based on lizard regrowth studies to grow his arm back, but was transformed into a human reptile. When the Lizard reverts back to human form, his reptilian arm returns to its amputated state.

1963: **The Chief with mobility issues** was created by Bob Haney, Arnold Drake, and Bruno Premiani of DC Comics (*My Greatest Adventure* #80). As leader of The Doom Patrol, inventor/genius Niles Caulder, also known as The Chief, built weapons into his wheelchair. As a crime fighter with paraplegia, he also taught others to accept those who were outcast by society.

1963: **Professor X with paraplegia** was created by Stan Lee and Jack Kirby of Marvel Comics (*X-Men* #1). Leading the X-Men from his wheelchair, Charles Xavier, also known as Professor X, fights for equal rights for mutants, when he's not battling super-villains.

1963: **Nick Fury with a visual impairment** was created by Stan Lee and Jack Kirby of Marvel Comics (*Sgt. Fury and his Howling Commandos* #1). During the war he was hit with shrapnel in one eye and eventually lost his sight in that eye. He began wearing a patch as a CIA agent and as an agent of the secret super-spy agency called SHIELD.

1963: **Iron Man with heart issues** was created by Stan Lee, Larry Lieber, Don Heck, and Jack Kirby of Marvel Comics (*Tales of Suspense* #39). Wearing magnetic armor to keep the shrapnel fragment lodged in his chest from reaching his heart, Iron Man's assistive technology is also great for thrashing bad guys.

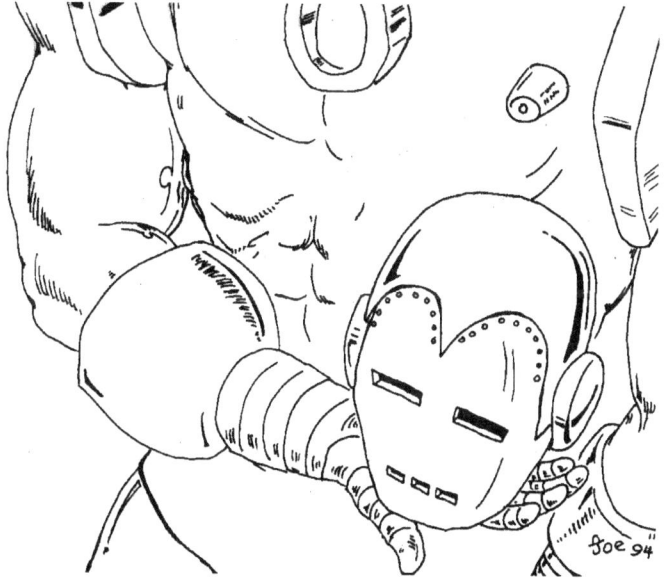

1964: **The Green Goblin with a mental illness** was created by Stan Lee and Steve Ditko of Marvel Comics (*Amazing Spider-Man* #14). Norman Osborn acquired a mental illness as a result of serum and a chemical explosion and became one of Spider-Man's most notorious villains.

1964: **Daredevil with blindness** was created by Stan Lee and Bill Everett of Marvel Comics (*Daredevil* #1). While loaded with many heightened senses, Matthew Murdock, also known as a Daredevil, is a crime-fighting lawyer who is totally blind.

1965: **Mr. Bailey with an undisclosed disability** was created by the Social Security Administration in *Three Who Came Back*. The third short story in this American public awareness comic book is called The End of a Dream. Therein, challenges for the Bailey family arise when Mr. Bailey's doctor declares that he "will never be able to work again." To the rescue comes cash disability benefits from Social Security. God bless America!

1969: Number One (Numero Uno) with mobility issues was created in Italy by Luciano Secchi and Roberto Raviola for the *Alan Ford* series. So old he claims to have known Homer, Number One uses a wheelchair and is the shrewd leader of Alan Ford and other members of a secret organization known as TNT.

1971: Black Racer is paralyzed from the neck down when in the human form of Willie Walker, a Vietnam veteran. Jack Kirby created this grim reaper type of character who travels about on cosmic-powered skis. Black Racer first appeared in *New Gods* #3 (DC Comics).

1976: Harvey Pekar with depression was the autobiographical writer of *American Splendor* (self-published).

1978: Many biblical people with disabilities are healed in *The Picture Bible* by Iva Hoth and Andre Le Blanc for Cook Communications. Among the many healed in this massive comic adaptation of the Bible include Naaman, a Syrian general with leprosy, which is a skin disease (from 2 Kings 5). The

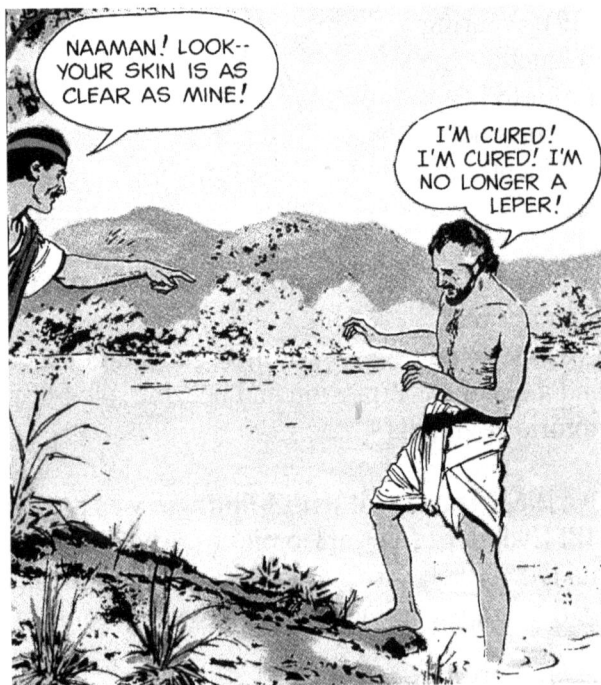

prophet Elisha tells Naaman to wash in the Jordan seven times. After a period of resistance and grumbling, Naaman finally does so and is "overcome with gratitude."

In the New Testament portion of *The Picture Bible*, Jesus also heals a large number of people, including a man with a withered hand, a man who couldn't walk and had to be let down through a hole in the roof, a girl on her death bed, and a man who was blind.

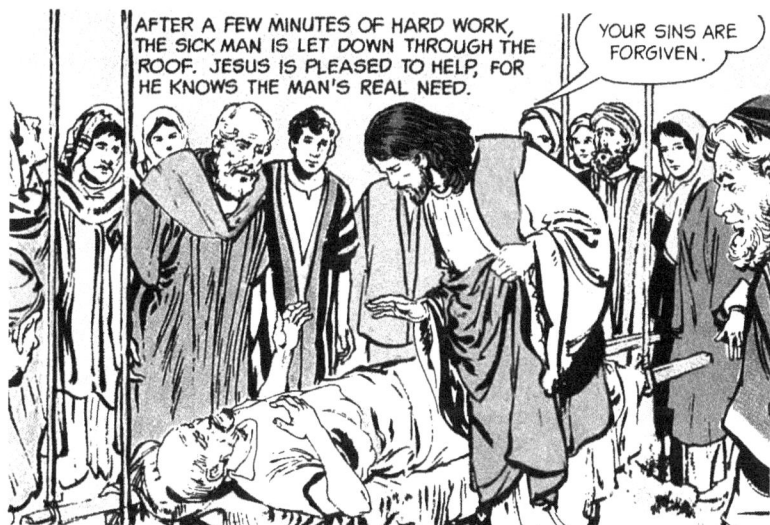

Another noteworthy person with a disability from *The Picture Bible* is the mighty Samson.

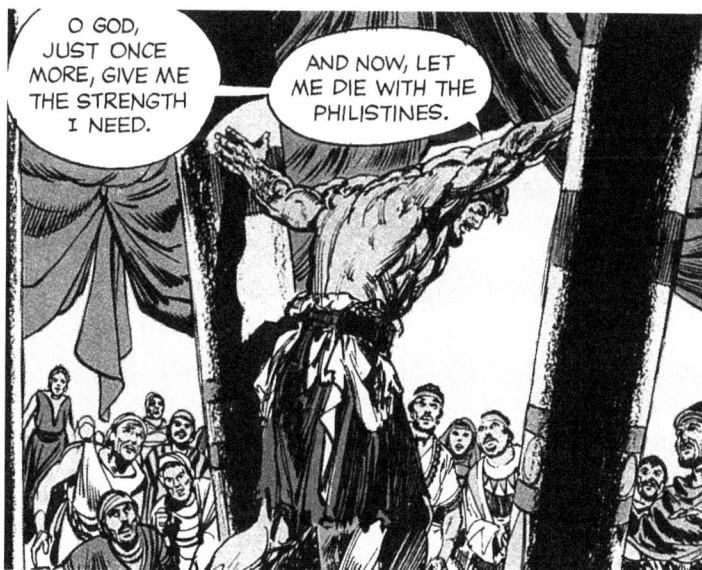

Near the end of his life, he was captured and blinded after being betrayed by the woman he loved: Delilah. Despite these grim circumstances, Samson's last act, as a man who was completely blind, was to defeat his lifelong enemies: the Philistines. Samson did so at the expense of his own life while also taking down plenty of Philistines as well as the Philistine temple to their false god, Dagon (adapted from Judges 16).

Samson has also appeared in numerous comic books over the years, including *A Spectacular Feature* #11 (1950 by Fox Features), and *Tales from the Great Book* #1 (1955 by Famous Funnies).

1983: **Puck as a person of short stature** was created by John Byrne of Marvel Comics (*Alpha Flight* #1). Eugene Judd is a great acrobat/fighter as Puck.

1980: **Cyborg with prosthetic limbs** was created by Marv Wolfman and George Perez of DC Comics (*DC Comics Presents* #26). After being severely mutilated in an alien-monster attack, Victor Stone is fitted with prosthetics over most of his body and becomes Cyborg. After a rough period of adjustment to his disability, he becomes a core member of the Teen Titans.

1985: **Leeder O. Men with paraplegia** was created by John Lytle and is the main character of the comic strip *dizABLED*. The character uses his wheelchair in all sorts of unique ways and speaks on disability issues.

1987: **The One-Arm Swordsman with a missing right arm** was published by Victory Comics. When Chan Lam lost his arm in a kung fu battle, he became a restaurant laborer (*One-Arm Swordsman* #1). Doing all his food service tasks with only one arm, he increased his strength and speed significantly. Needless to say, when trouble arises, the One-Arm Swordsman will be ready.

1989: **Batgirl became The Oracle with paraplegia** in a plot by writer John Ostrander and editor Kim Yale of DC Comics (*Suicide Squad* #23). After Barbara Gordon was shot by the Joker and became a person with paraplegia, she began using her detective skills to help other heroes fight crime--all from her wheelchair.

1993: **Joe Chiappetta with chronic back pain** slowly starts to introduce his disability issues into the auto-biographical *Silly Daddy* comic series (reprinted in the *Silly Daddy* 2004 graphic novel). Chiappetta was first mentioned as a person with back pain in the second issue of *Silly Daddy* (1993). By *Silly Daddy* #19 in 1998, the years of being a road warrior, driving around to comic book conventions, had finally gotten the best of him; he was full of

My spinal branch wasn't made to sit still for so long. This berry cream that my ex-girlfriend Deniberry left me should help a little.

tension and rubbing pain relief medicine on his aching back while cruising through the interstate highway in search of cartoon glory.

1993: **Batman acquired a spinal cord injury** in *Batman* #497 by Doug Moench and Jim Aparo (DC Comics). Bane, a steroid-enhanced villain gave Batman this disability at a ruthless Batcave battle. In a multi-issue story arc, he went through rehabilitation and was paranormally healed, leaving his wheelchair behind.

1994: **Harvey Pekar with cancer** (lymphoma) was a main character in *Our Cancer Year* published by Four Walls Eight Windows. It's a true story/graphic novel by Harvey Pekar, Joyce Brabner and Frank Stack.

1995: **John Porcellino with hyperacusis** (hypersensitivity to sound) was first disclosed as John's disability in his autobiographical *King-Cat* #48 from June of 1995, the same year he acquired the disability. John covered his experience with hyperacusis in more detail for his graphic novel, *Diary of a Mosquito Abatement Man*, published by La Mano in 2005.

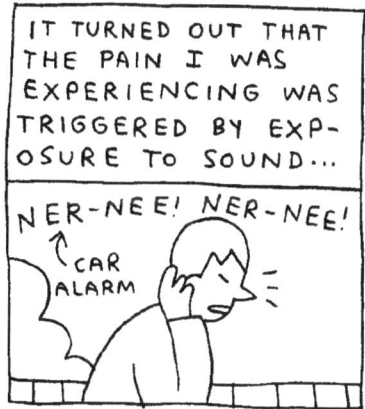

1998: **Spider-Man from an alternate universe with an amputation** is created by Tom DeFalco and Ronald Frenz of Marvel Comics (*What If...* #105). In the MC2 alternate universe, Spider-Man lost his leg in battle and uses an artificial leg.

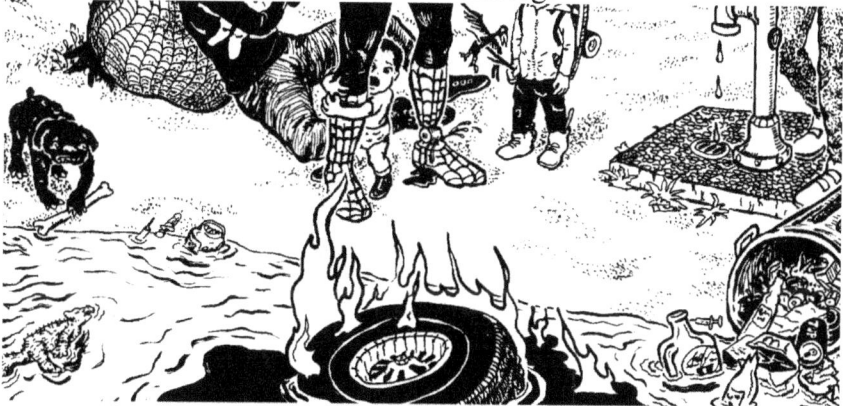

Personal artistic side note: Ironically enough, in 1993 I drew a character called Svider-Man with an artificial foot that was leaking oil. The drawing was concept art that doubled as social commentary. This was during my "mad at the world, life is unfair, rebel" stage of life.

1999: **Echo with deafness** was created by David Mack and Joe Quesada of Marvel Comics (*Daredevil*, vol. 2, #9). Maya Lopez, also known as Echo, is deaf and a great fighter with photographic reflexes.

2003: **David Karasik with autism** was a main character in *The Ride Together*. It's a graphic novel created by Paul and Judy Karasik for Washington Square Press. The book is a brother and sister's account of life with their brother, David, who has autism.

2004: **Shannon Lake with an intellectual disability** was created by Lynn Johnston as a minor character in the comic strip *For Better or for Worse*. Introduced into the comic as a person with an intellectual disability, Shannon helped to educate more readers about social communication challenges.

2004: **Seth Torres with autism** was a boy created by Karen Montague-Reyes for the comic strip *Clear Blue Water*. The cartoonist draws a fictional family with five kids (one being Seth) and pulls from her real life experience as a mother of five children. One of her kids is severely autistic.

2005: **Jean-Christophe Beauchard with epilepsy** was a main character in *Epileptic*. It's a graphic novel created by David Beauchard for Pantheon Books. The cartoonist's brother, Jean-Christophe, has severe grand mal seizures, and family life with epilepsy is covered extensively. This autobiography was originally serialized in French beginning in 1996.

2006: **Marisa Acocella Marchetto with breast cancer** was the main character of her autobiographical graphic novel *Cancer Vixen: A True Story* published by Pantheon.

2011: **Tyler Page with attention deficit disorder** created his autobiographical account about living with ADD in his webcomic *Raised on Ritalin*.

Lessons Learned from Disability in Comics

After much study of characters with disabilities in the history of comics, a number of patterns come to light. Disability is rarely the central theme in comics, yet since health problems are a part of life, instances of disability continue to pepper the comics of every century wherein sequential arts are found. When persons with disabilities are depicted as little more than a convenient plot device, disability is usually--but not always--portrayed with negative or pitiful stereotypes and misconceptions about persons with disabilities.

Nevertheless, instances of health impairments as central themes in comics seem to be slowly, yet steadily, increasing. This is especially noticeable in the later half of the 20th century. However, no single character or creator can be credited as the sole driver of this trend. The more personal experience any creator has with disability issues, the more likely his or her work will reflect proper and respectful attitudes toward persons with disabilities.

As the decentralization of publishing continues through the digital age, more and more persons with disabilities will continue to create nontraditional comics focused on disability. These works will reflect a worldview that captures life with disability more accurately, and with a greater degree of relatability as well as inspiration.

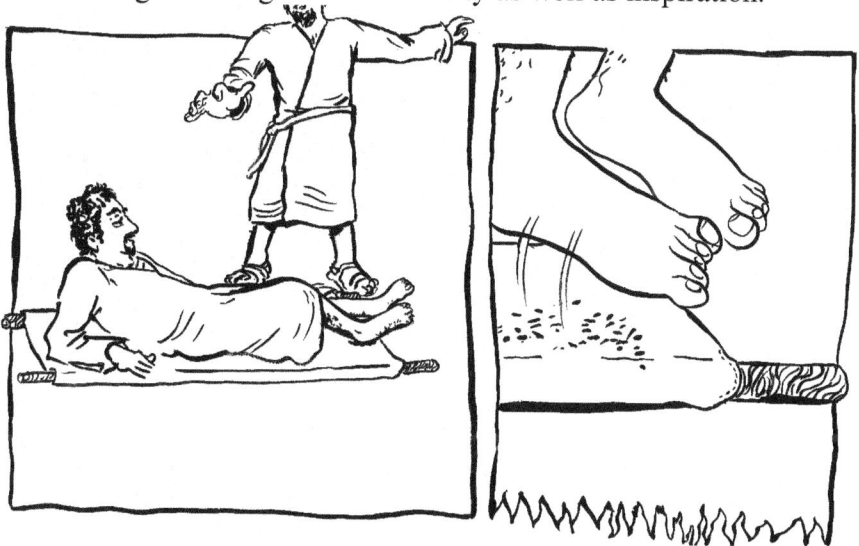

Maria Chiappetta

On Being a Daughter of Silly Daddy

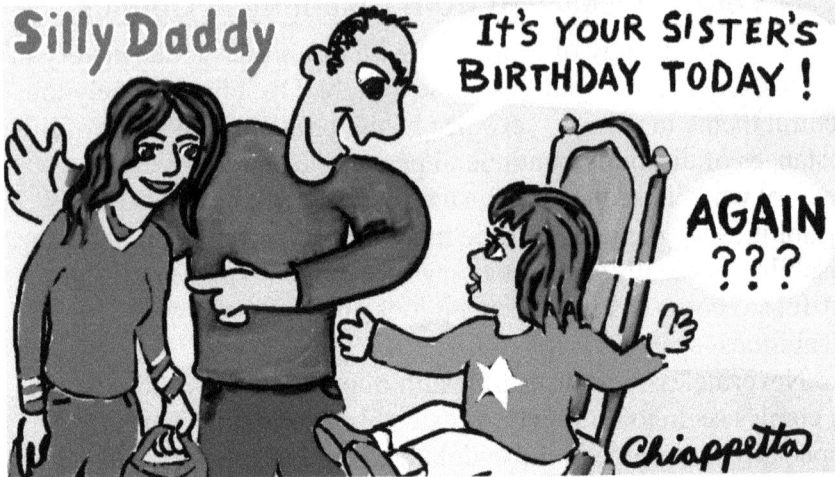

Having daughters is one of the most amazing components of my entire life. I am honored to publish the following article written by my oldest daughter Maria.

Growing Up Silly Daddy: A Silly Daughter Report

In the autumn of 2011, my dad approached me about writing a piece for the 20th anniversary of his comic, *Silly Daddy*. Let me just put a cheap disclaimer on this by saying I am not cut out for writing. My thoughts wander and overlap, and it is often hard to translate them into cohesive sentences.

I hadn't read *Silly Daddy* as an "adult" until about a year or two ago. Of course I had seen it throughout the years, but reading it at an older age was certainly different. Honestly, it was a bittersweet read. I remember being bored one night in my '70s puke-green room (a color I excitedly picked...), pulling out the graphic novel, and crying a lot. I felt as if I shouldn't be reading it. Most kids don't see their parent's firsthand account of their divorce, parenting troubles, and dating life. My heart broke for my young father and mother, only a little older than I am now, trying to raise me, keep the family together, and attempting to have social lives/careers of their own. It made me fearful of my own future. Would I be able to have a lasting relationship? Would I be a decent parent one day? It raised a lot of questions in me, not to mention made me wonder what other kids featured in autobio/diary comics would think one day. From James

Kochalka's *American Elf* comics, what will Eli and Oliver Kochalka think of one day? More relevantly, what will Luke and Anna Chiappetta think one day?

Ultimately, though, *Silly Daddy* makes me grin. In it I see most of my current personality traits, likes and dislikes; my disdain for big chains, love of the woods, bike-riding, granola, and deeply rooted sentimentality and introspection. One of my favorite quotes, from the 1985 Marvel comic *Kitty Pryde and Wolverine* #3 (written by Chris Claremont), could easily be an early *Silly Daddy* monologue:

"I hate cities...hate civilization, with all its idiot rules. Gimme the free, open, elemental spaces of my mountains where a man holds his fate in his own hands. No lies there, no deception, no compromise."

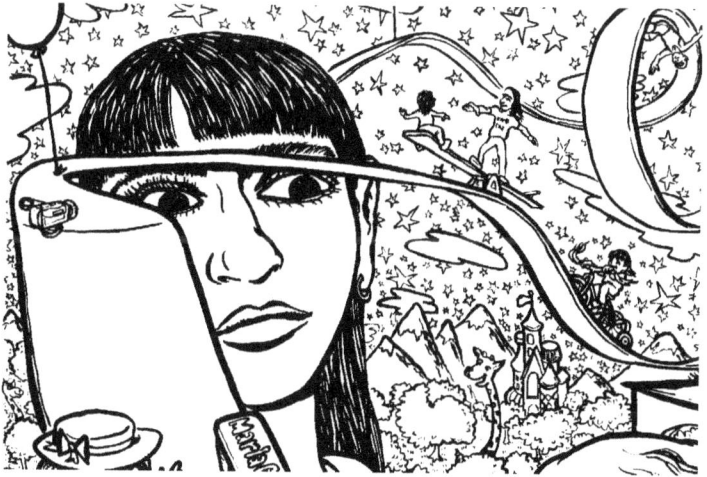

It is incredible to see how much my dad has shaped me. Also, on a slightly unrelated note, it kind of weirds me out to see how much I look like what he thought I would (see "A Death in the Family" from *Silly Daddy* 2004 graphic novel.)

Finally, it is amazing to see how much my dad has changed. I got to know him both as a hippieish cartoonist as a young child, and as a Christian as a kid/young adult. He is now one of the most patient, insightful people I know. I've heard him say that some of his original fans may have dropped him when he became a Christian, but I wish they could look past their religious-phobias and see him as I've come to know him. Today there are so many empty comics, dark for the sake of being dark. *Silly Daddy* is not one of them. It remains funny, serious, deep, and sometimes cheesy, in the best way possible. My dad is still a talented artist, deep thinker, granola eater, and outside dweller. He's still a Silly Daddy. Happy 20th, *Silly Daddy*!

Maria Chiappetta, 2011

Silly Daddy 20th Anniversary Comics

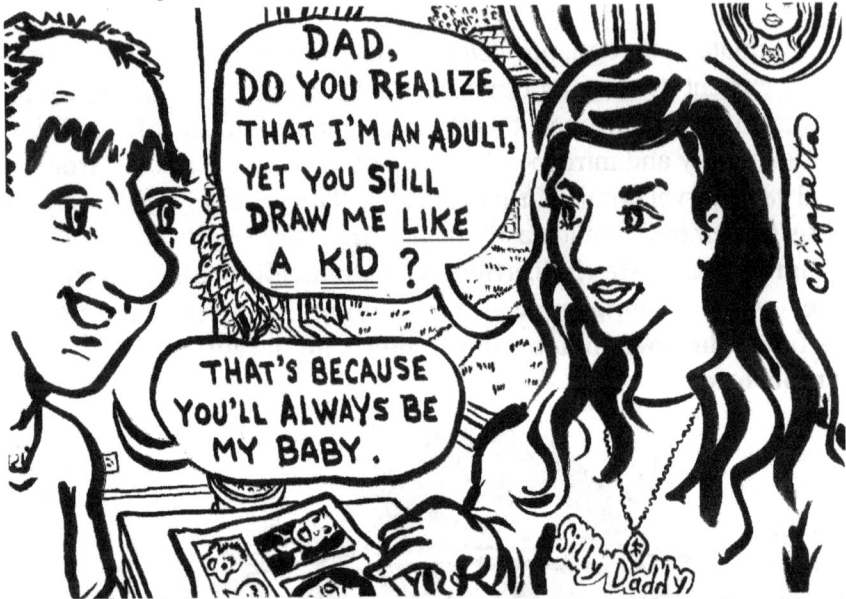

To celebrate 20 years of *Silly Daddy* comics, please enjoy this bonus cartoon section featuring some of my favorite scenes with my favorite peoples. Before I became a father, thinking like a parent was totally foreign to me, yet now, I can't imagine any other mindset.

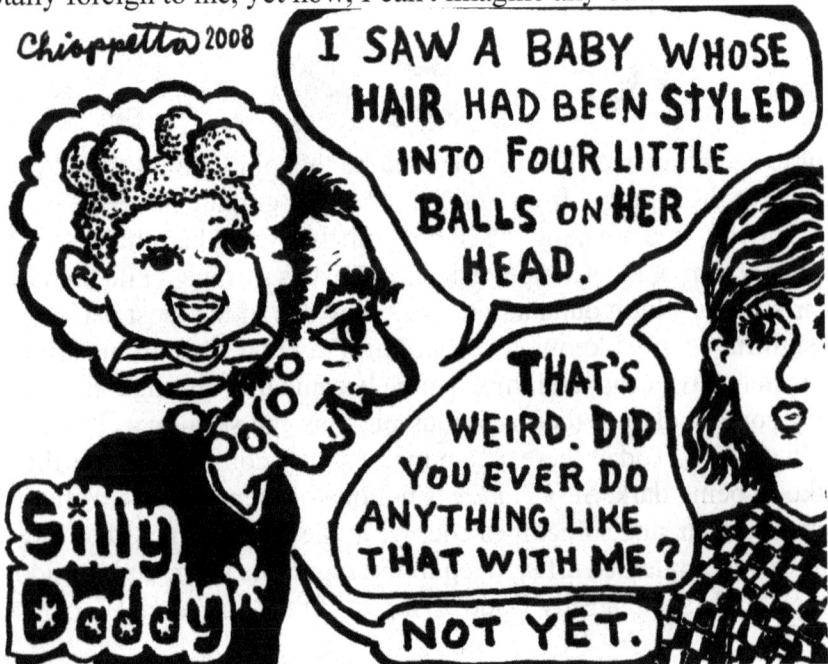

If you are not a parent and you have a hard time understanding the full depth of this comic, or the amazing essay that my daughter Maria wrote, the 1991 remake movie *Father of the Bride* starring Steve Martin does an excellent job at making fatherhood real and appealing for the masses. My hope, of course, as an author, is that I too can share fun, family, and faithful truths with you as a Silly Daddy!

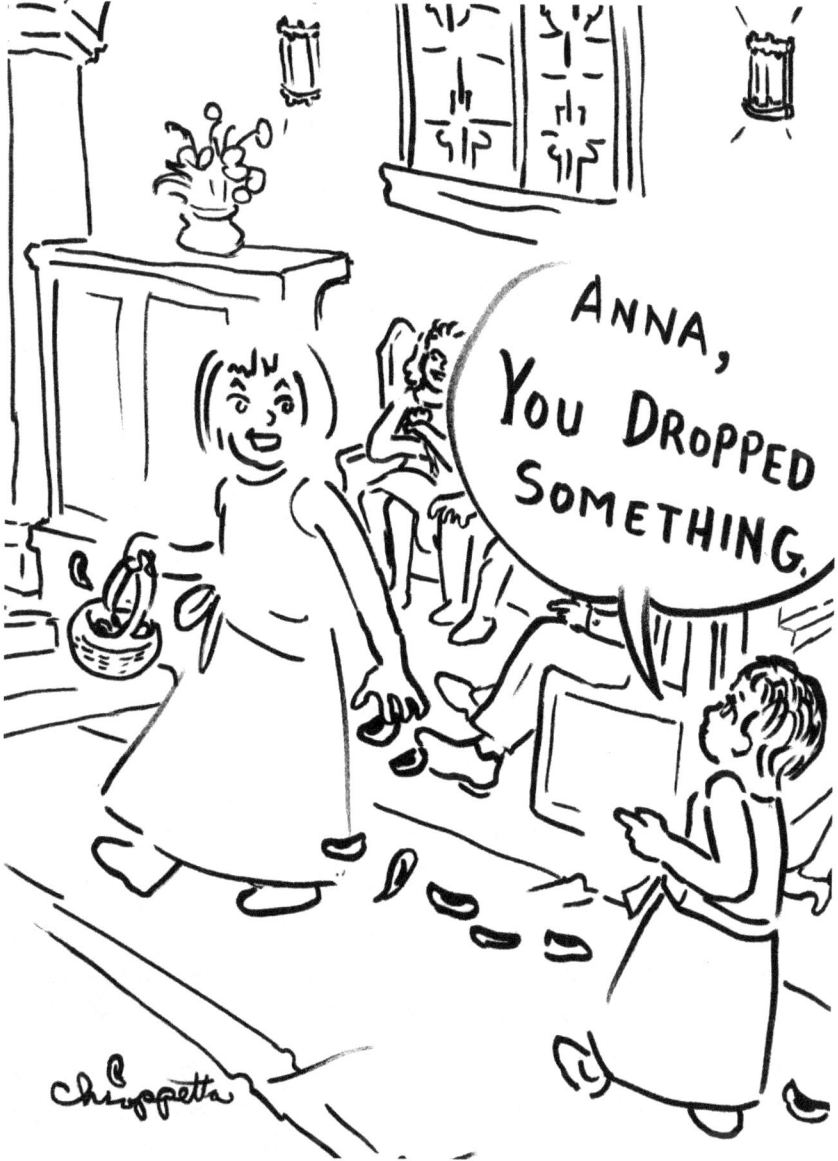

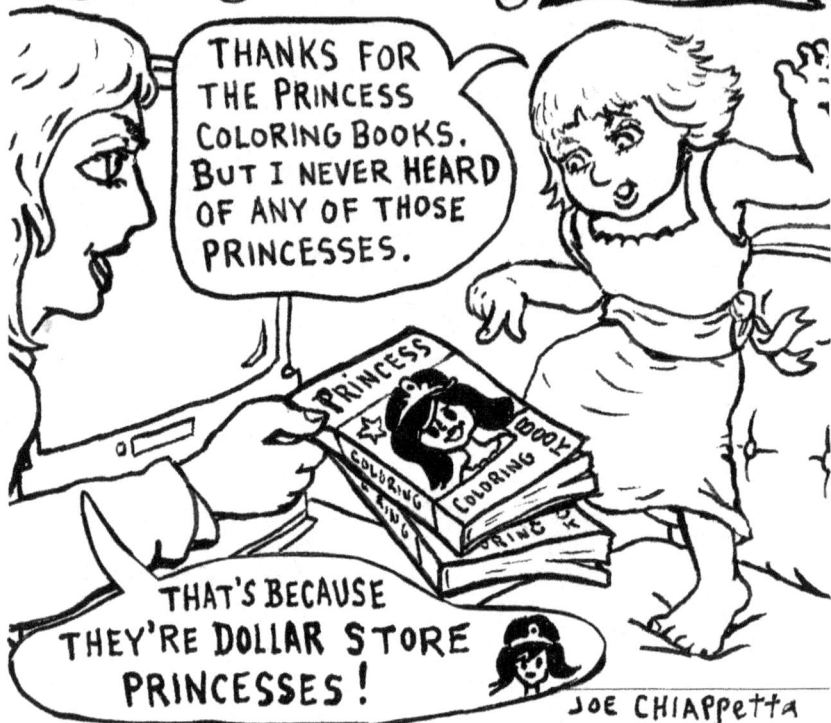

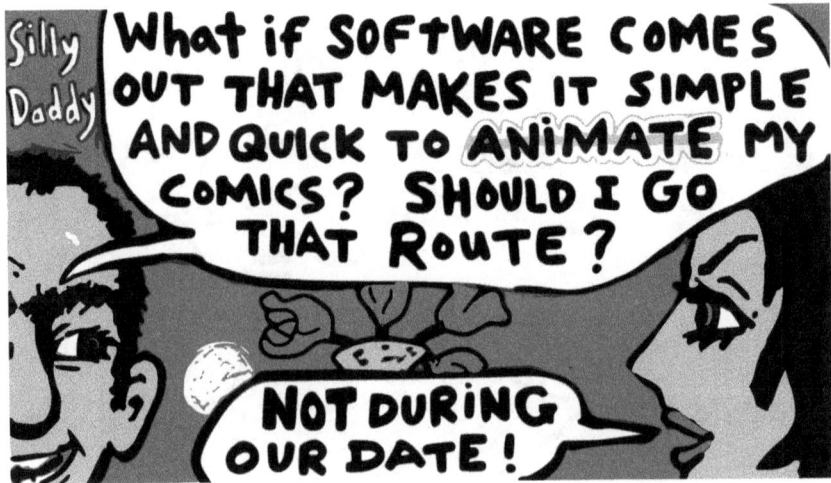

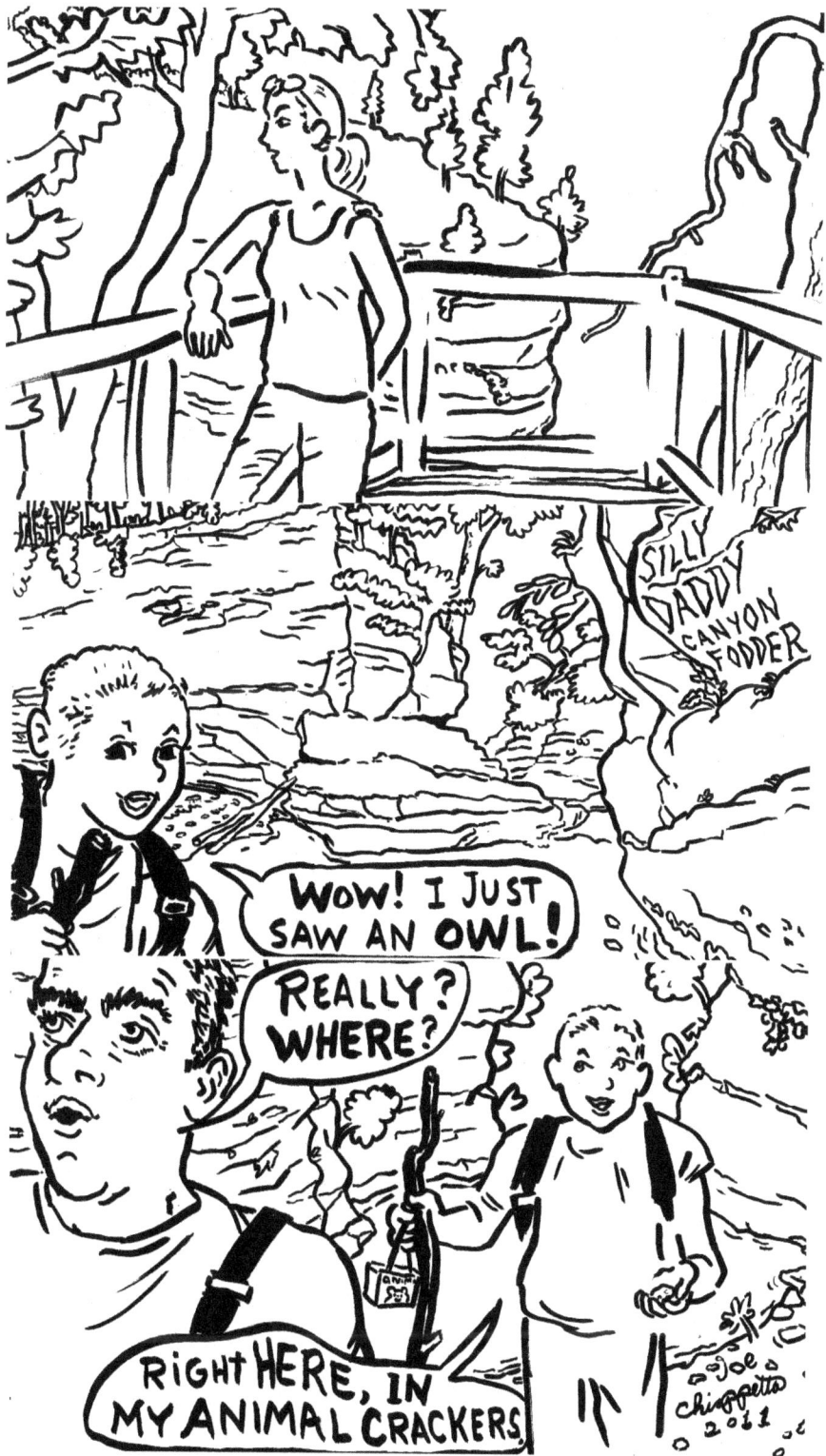

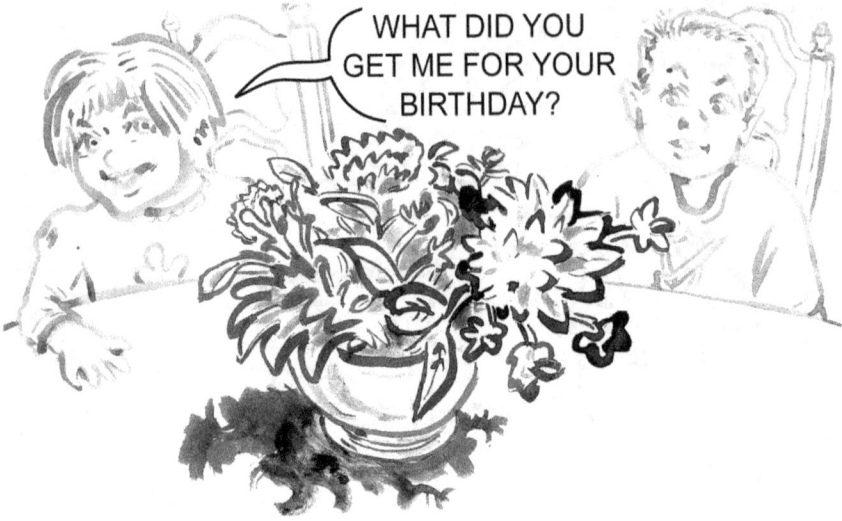

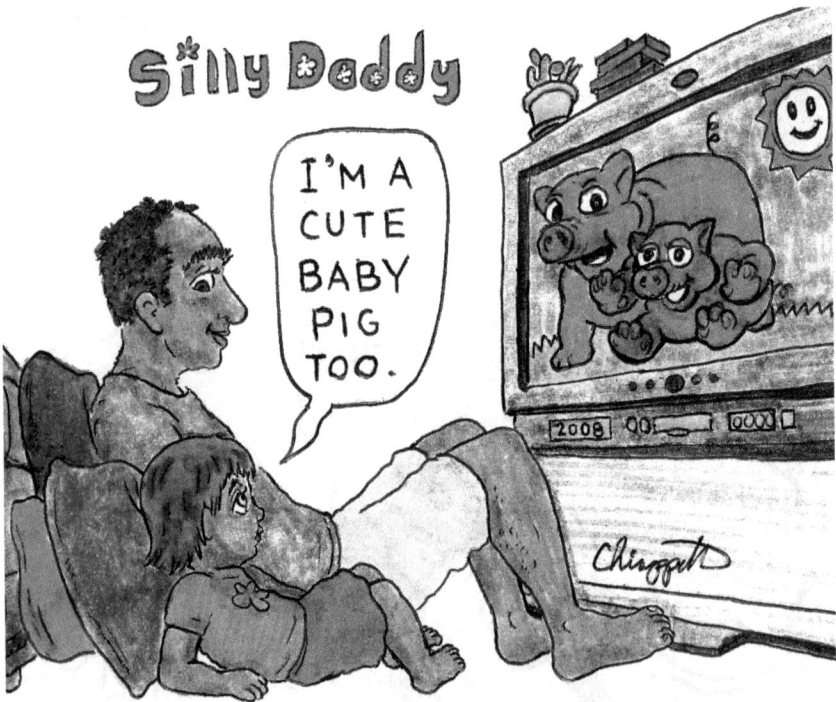

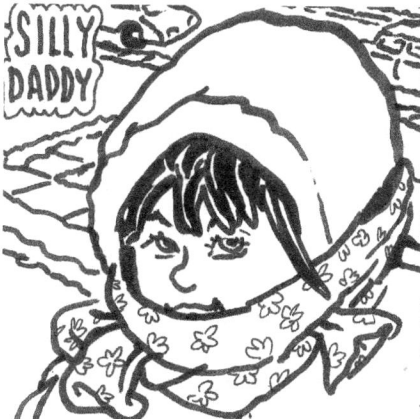

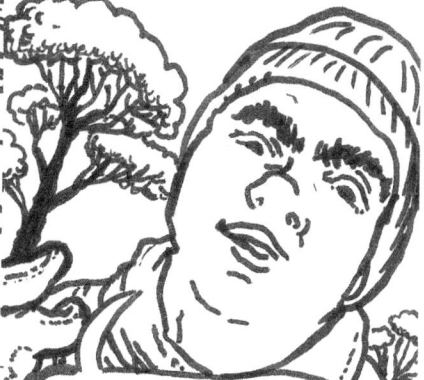

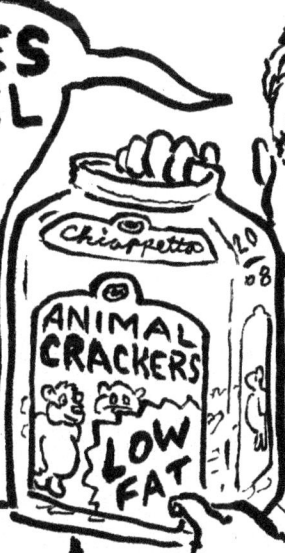

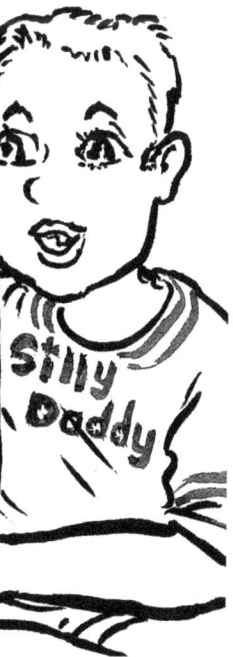

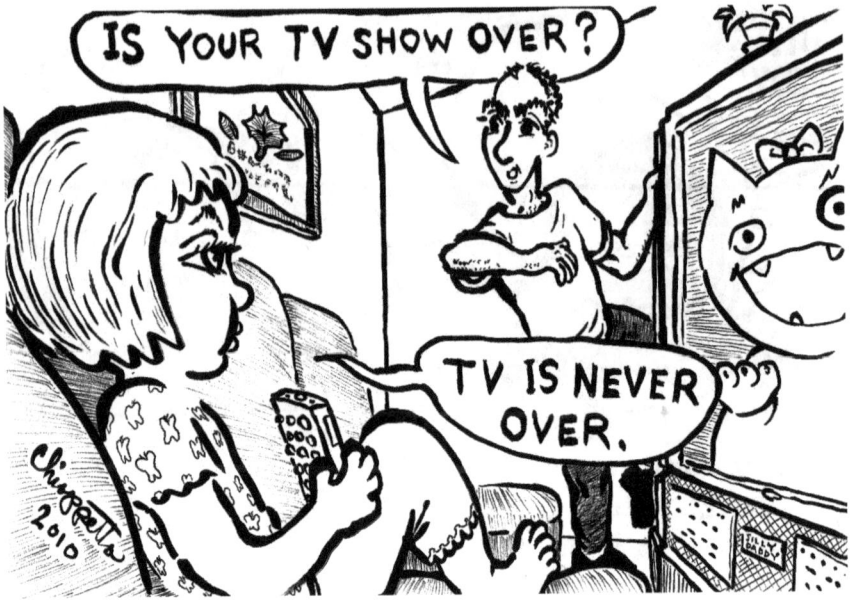

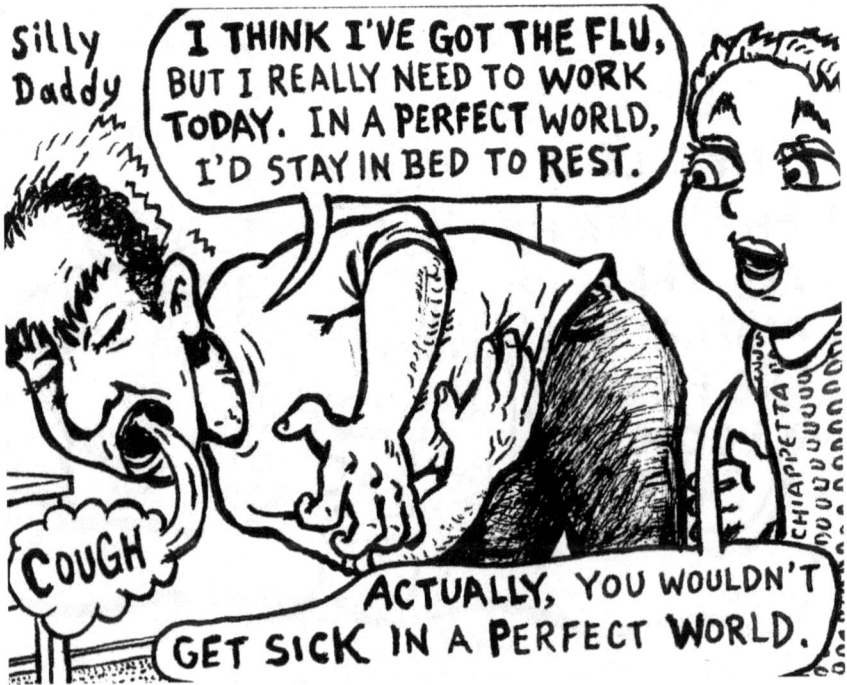

Joe Chiappetta

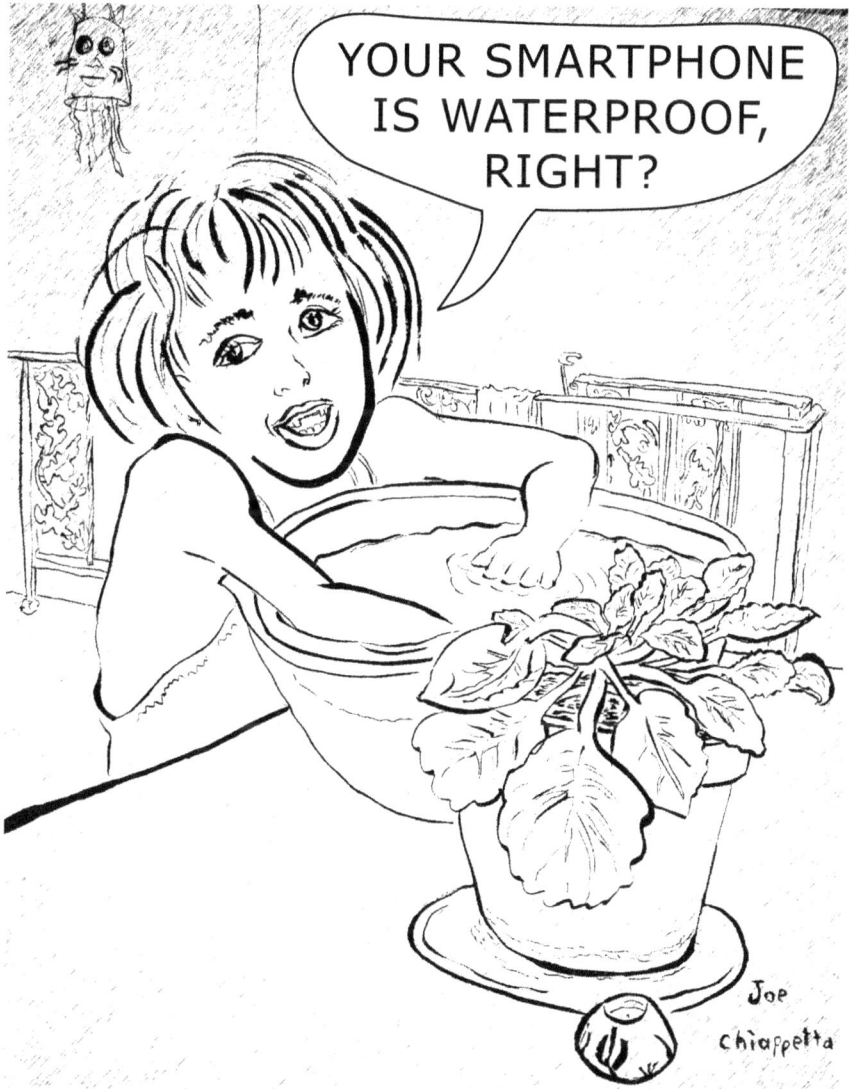

SILLY DADDY...
Die-Hard Writer

WHAT IF I INVENTED A MACHINE THAT COPIED YOUR INTELLECT SO WELL, THAT IT COULD WRITE BOOKS *AS IF* THEY CAME FROM YOUR OWN MIND? WOULD YOU STILL WRITE YOUR *OWN* BOOKS?

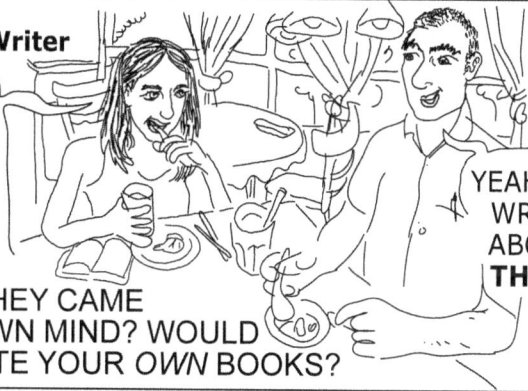

YEAH, I'D WRITE ABOUT **THAT**.

Silly Daddy Romance

My wife and I went on a walk in the woods for our date.

CHIAPPETTA 2007

LOOK! THERE'S THE TENT OF A HOMELESS GUY.

LET'S GO BY THE RIVER.

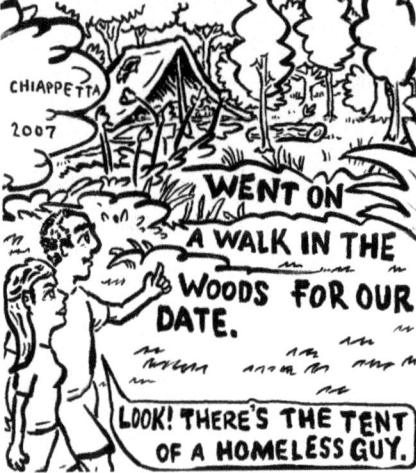

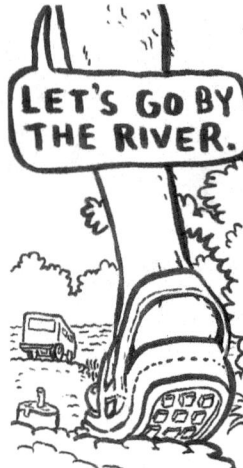

ASIDE FROM THE USUAL NATURE STUFF, WE ALSO SAW SIGNS OF FRINGE CIVILIZATION INCLUDING A PERSON LIVING IN THEIR VAN, VOODOO BEADS WITH A CANDLE, PLUS THAT HOMELESS GUY.

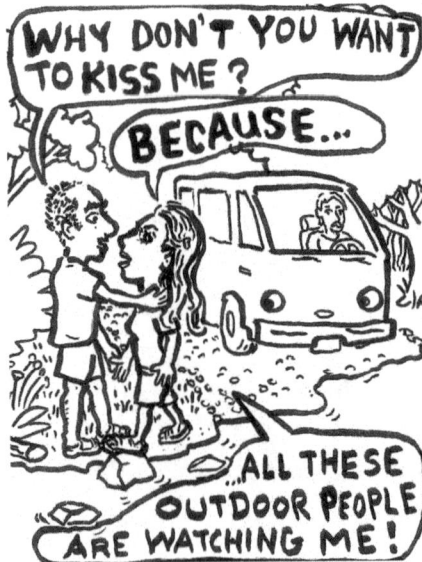

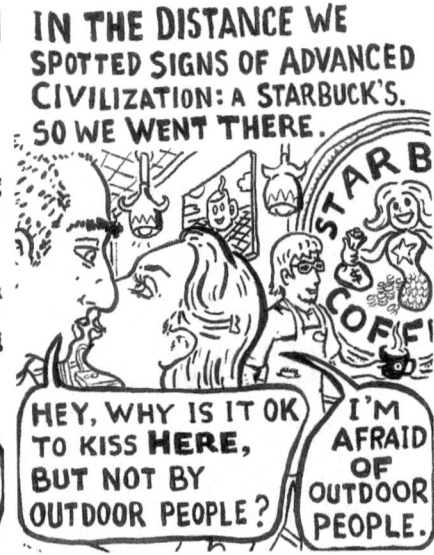

WHY DON'T YOU WANT TO KISS ME?

BECAUSE...

...ALL THESE OUTDOOR PEOPLE ARE WATCHING ME!

IN THE DISTANCE WE SPOTTED SIGNS OF ADVANCED CIVILIZATION: A STARBUCK'S. SO WE WENT THERE.

HEY, WHY IS IT OK TO KISS **HERE**, BUT NOT BY OUTDOOR PEOPLE?

I'M AFRAID OF OUTDOOR PEOPLE.

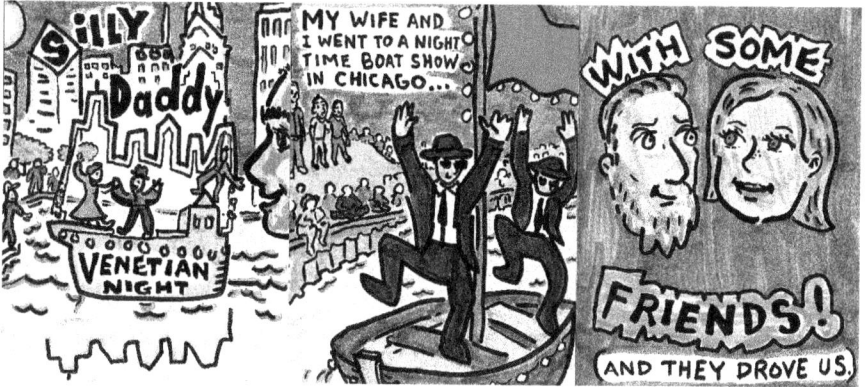

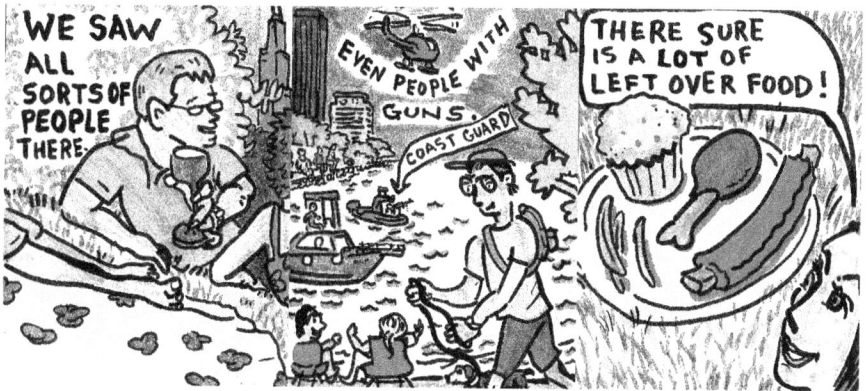

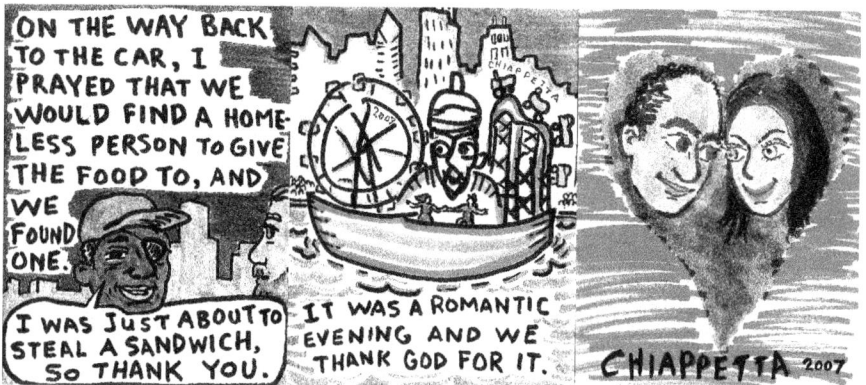

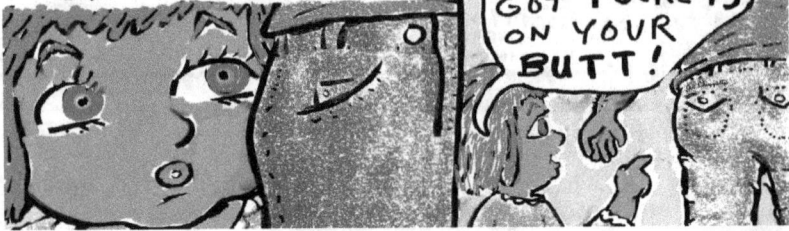

MOST PAIRS OF TODDLER PANTS ONLY HAVE POCKETS IN THE FRONT. THIS PROMPTED MY 3 YEAR OLD TO DISCOVER...

HEY! YOU'VE GOT POCKETS ON YOUR BUTT!

SILLY DADDY

COURAGE

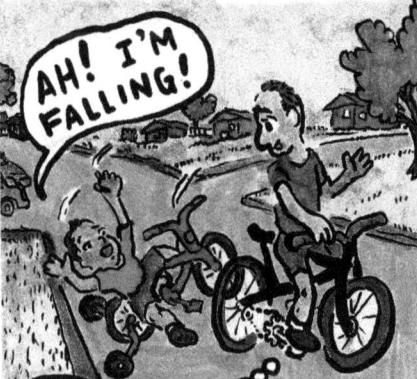

AH! I'M FALLING!

HE'S FALLING SO SLOWLY. I'M SURE HE CAN'T BE HURT.

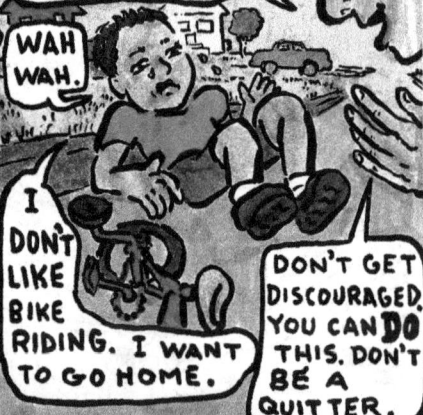

YOU'RE OKAY, SON. JUST GET BACK ON THE BIKE. LET'S KEEP RIDING.

WAH WAH.

I DON'T LIKE BIKE RIDING. I WANT TO GO HOME.

DON'T GET DISCOURAGED. YOU CAN DO THIS. DON'T BE A QUITTER.

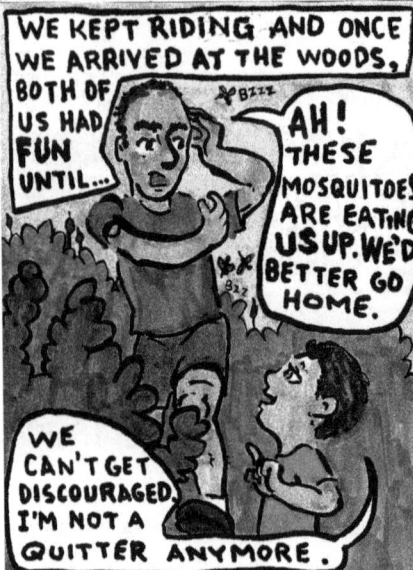

WE KEPT RIDING AND ONCE WE ARRIVED AT THE WOODS, BOTH OF US HAD FUN UNTIL...

BZZ

AH! THESE MOSQUITOES ARE EATING US UP. WE'D BETTER GO HOME.

WE CAN'T GET DISCOURAGED. I'M NOT A QUITTER ANYMORE.

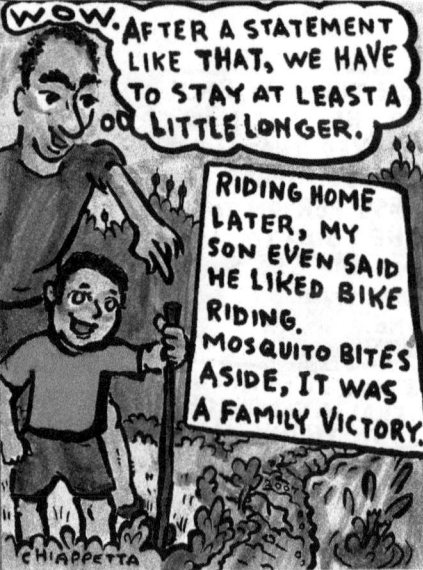

WOW. AFTER A STATEMENT LIKE THAT, WE HAVE TO STAY AT LEAST A LITTLE LONGER.

RIDING HOME LATER, MY SON EVEN SAID HE LIKED BIKE RIDING. MOSQUITO BITES ASIDE, IT WAS A FAMILY VICTORY.

CHIAPPETTA

CIVIL WAR at the CIVIL WAR REENACTMENT

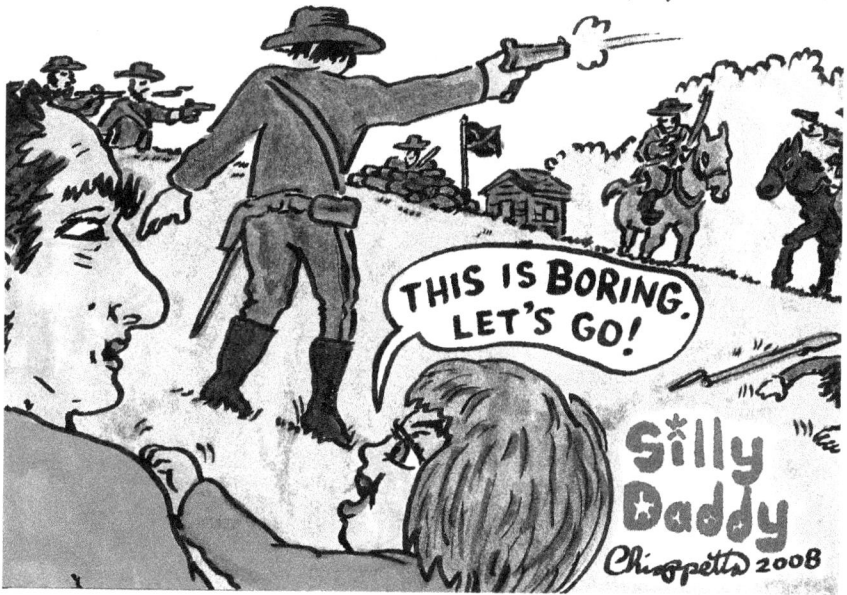

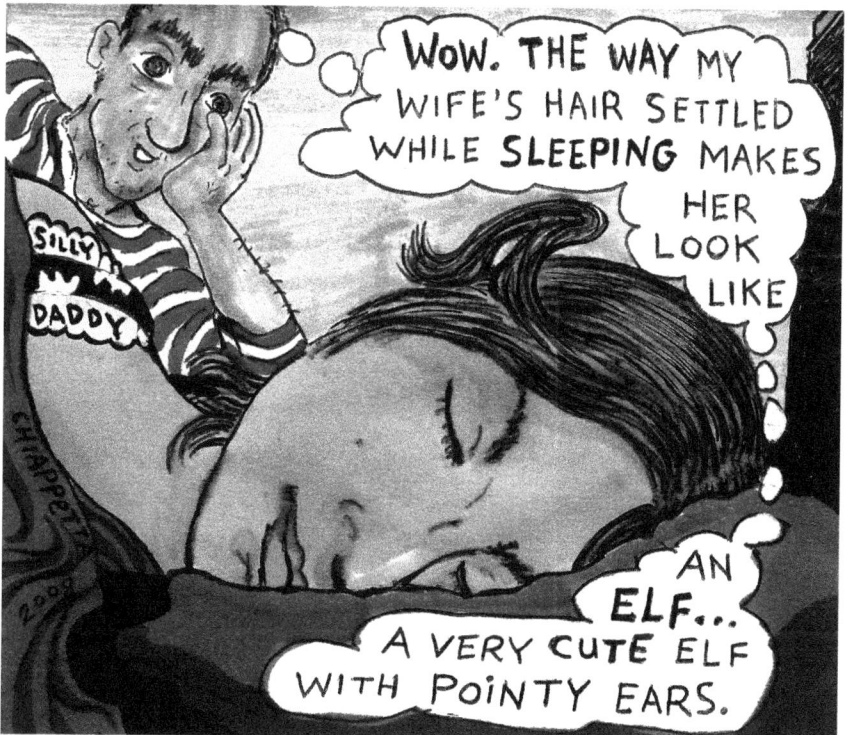

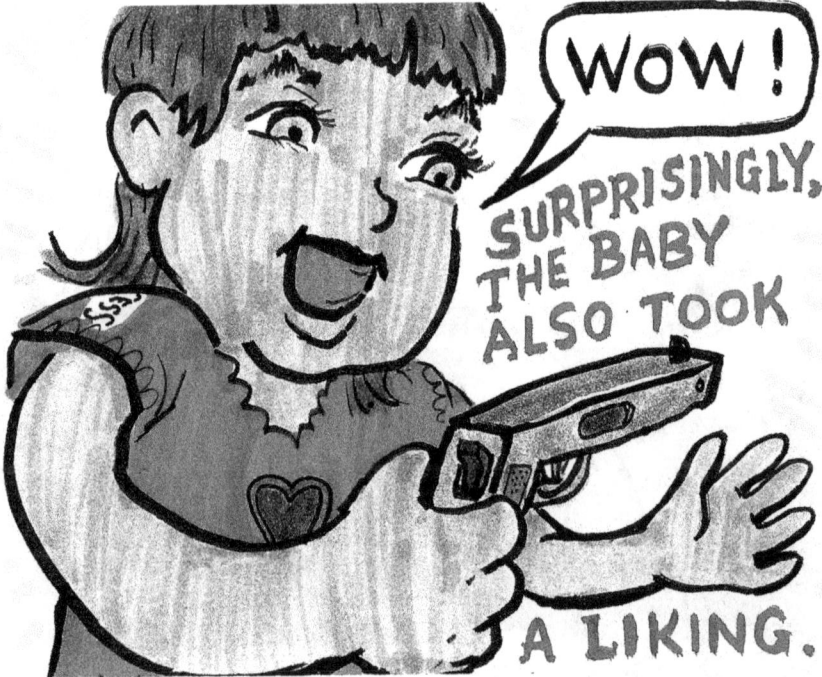

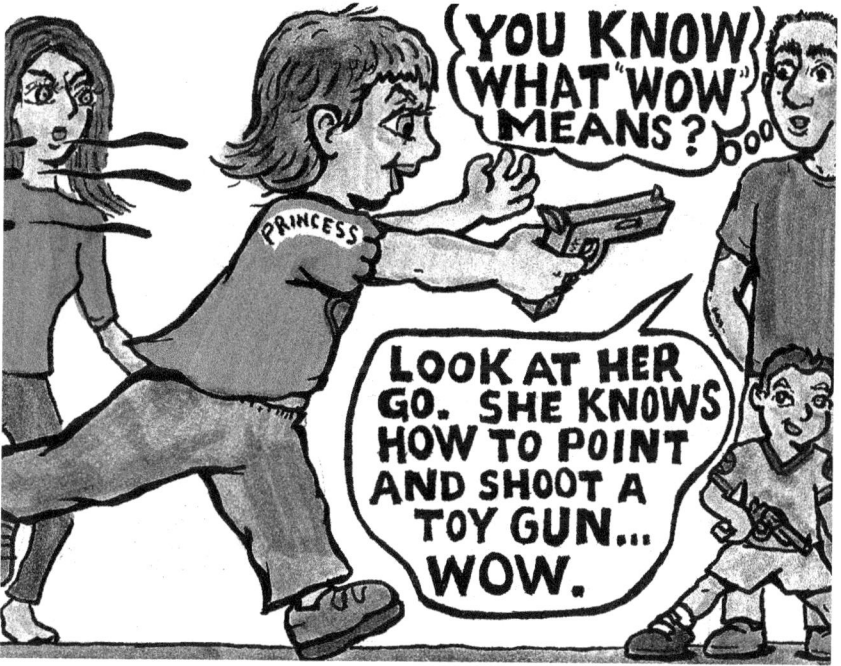

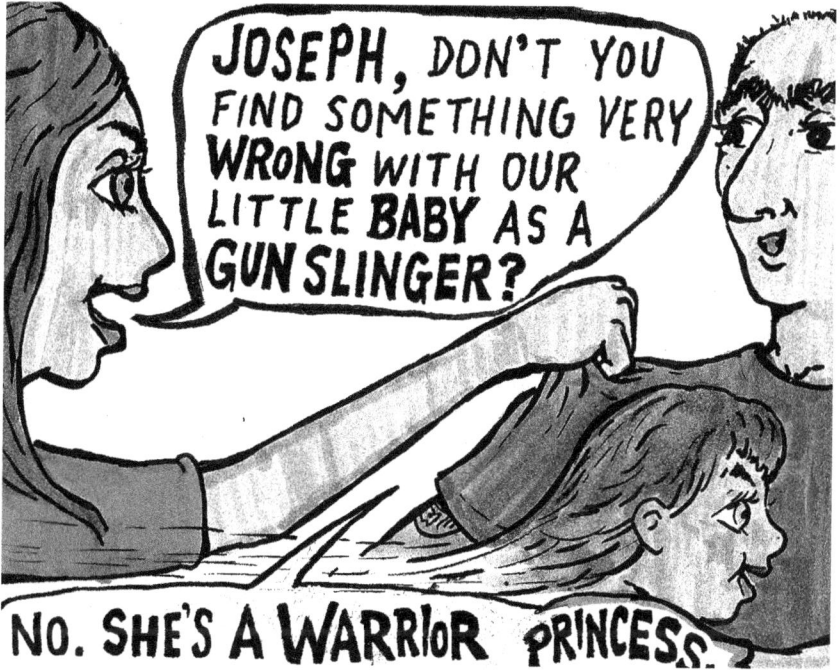

About the Author

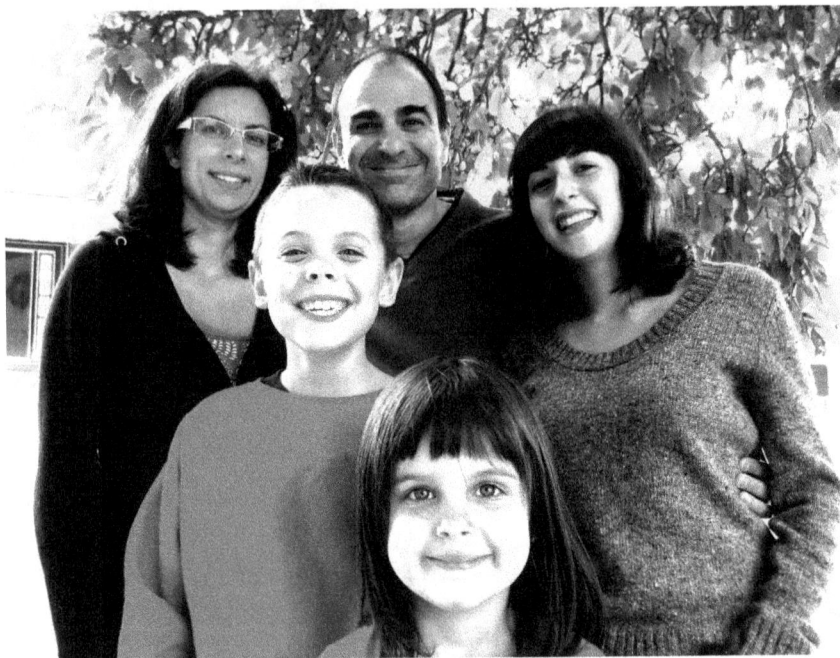

Joe Chiappetta is an American author and cartoonist, grateful to be happily married with three children. Currently living in North Riverside, Illinois, his formal education was from Northern Illinois University, where he received a Bachelor of Fine Arts, with an emphasis in painting.

While trained in the more traditional visual arts, his lifetime creative focus has been in writing and cartooning. As one of the key members of the Independent Comics Movement of the late 1980s and 1990s, Chiappetta's work is respected around the globe. He is best known as the man behind one of the longest-running autobiographical comics, *Silly Daddy*, which has been a rewarding creative endeavor since 1991. The series has received the following professional recognition:

- Xeric Award Winner
- Ignatz Award Nominee for Outstanding Story
- Harvey Award Nominee for Best New Series

While the bulk of Chiappetta's work has been within autobiographical comics, he has also maintained a focus on science fiction writing. *Silly Daddy* plots are notorious for taking off on sci-fi themed subplots. As a natural progression, Joe's 2010 release, *Star Chosen*, is a science fiction space opera for the whole family. That book was his first full-length novel without pictures.

In 1998 Joe became a Christian, which is often evident in the more hopeful world-view represented in his writings and comics thereafter. Due to personal experience with a number of health impairments, Joe also writes about disability issues in his work, combining humor with the intent to help others have more compassion for those in need. Living life to the full despite health challenges is a recurring theme in his stories. For his work on *The Back Pain Avenger*, Joe won an Illinois Arts Council award in 2012.

At a moment's notice, Joe is usually up for a good game of chess, bike-riding, building forts in the woods, wrestling, foam sword fighting, or Bible study. From his stories, one can tell that he enjoys spending time with God, family, other people with disabilities, science fiction geeks, and corny jokers.

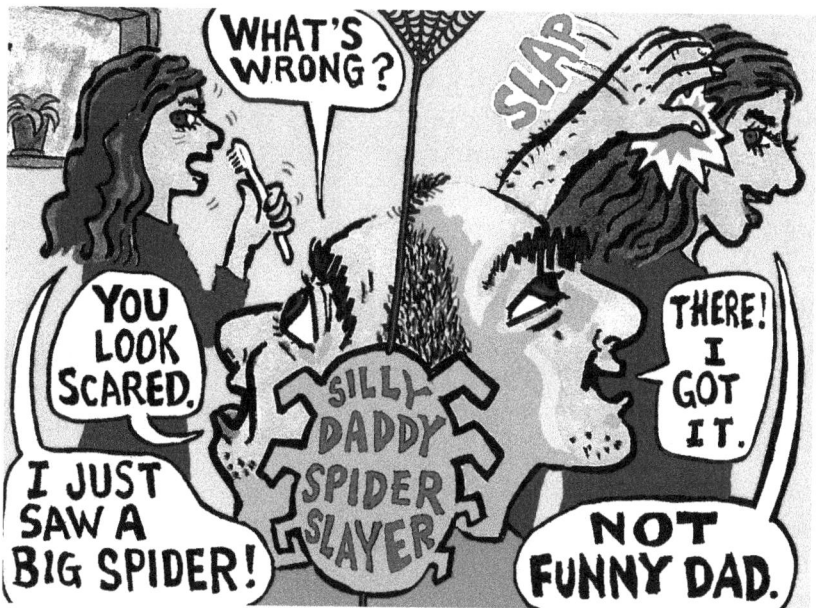

Catalog of Books by Chiappetta

Star Chosen: a science fiction novel
By Joe Chiappetta 2010

Think "Star Trek" meets the Bible. Deleting history was just the beginning. Blast off with STAR CHOSEN, a space opera of post-biblical proportions! After war, heartbreak, attacks to your faith, and the erasure of all history, whose side will you fight on: the Proud... or the Chosen? 67,000 words

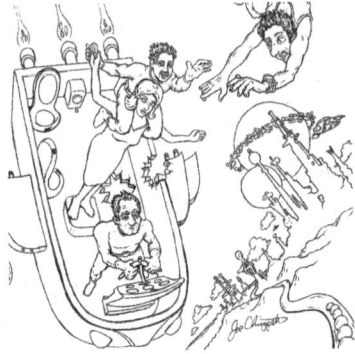

Power Pendant of Planet Pizon:
Star Chosen sci-fi novelette (eBook)

The Star Chosen are caught in a deadly struggle over a mysterious power pendant that may be the only thing standing between them and certain vaporization. When control over this otherworldly pendant gets called into controversy, a young romance on Planet Pizon turns into a fatal battle involving laser guns, spaceships, and ex-boyfriends. Short story contains 10,000 words.

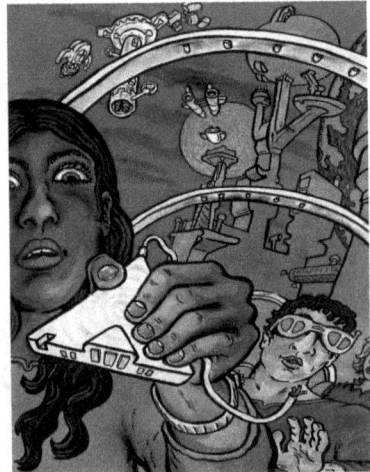

Armed with Intergalactic Weapons
(sci-fi illustrated eBook)

Autobiographical story of how a space boy becomes a fighter and an artist--on the wrong and right sides in the galactic battle between good and evil. 13,300 words with 42 illustrations

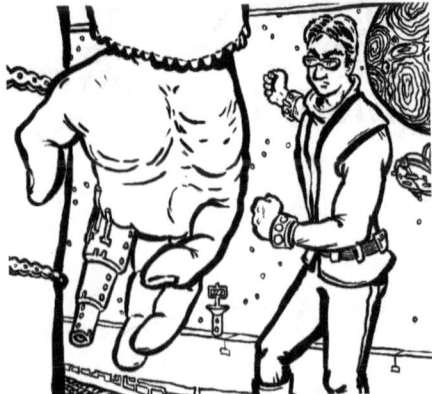

Silly Daddy in Space
Comic book (eBook)

It's sci-fi satire safe for all ages and androids too! Inside jokes and parodies abound for fans of Star Wars, Battlestar Galactica, and Star Trek. The colorful cast of offworld characters includes Office Space Girl, Christian Robot, funny and weird aliens, plus the whole family. 72 comics and illustrations plus 12,000 word cartoonist commentary

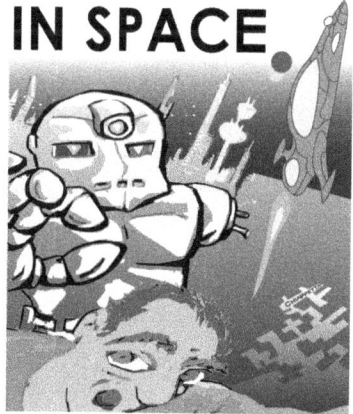

SILLY DADDY IN SPACE

Debt-Busters:
How to get out of debt using spiritual truths, not cheap gimmicks (eBook)

See what the Bible says about debt in this practical, helpful, and even funny how to get out of debt guide. If you are in financial debt or just want help managing money from a spiritual perspective, this is for you. Contains 7,000 words with 25 comics and illustrations

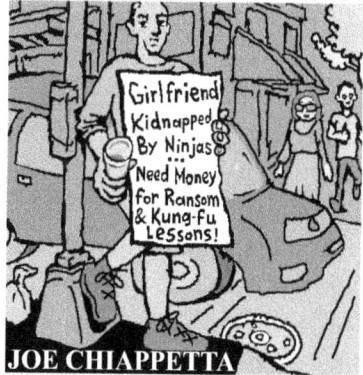

DEBT-BUSTERS

JOE CHIAPPETTA
How to get out of debt using Spiritual truths, not cheap gimmicks

Crucified Comics (eBook)
Go beyond a cartoon view of the cross with comics and spiritual commentary aimed to inspire personal accountability for what happened to Jesus at the crucifixion. This mix of comic book and text narrative has plenty of practical lessons for your quiet times with God as well as memorable and original images of Christianity today. Contains 10,000 words plus 68 comics and illustrations

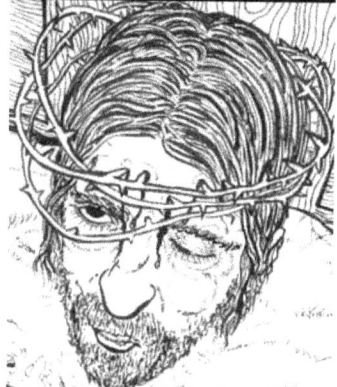

CRUCIFIED

COMICS

Genesis Jam: An Anthology Inspired by the Ultimate Creator (eBook)

Creative writers and artists striving to love God embrace the powerful themes of Genesis: good and evil, brotherhood, family, trust in God, mercy, and love. The Garden of Eden and Cain and Abel are the subjects of this faithful anthology. Works of fiction inspired by events in Genesis as well as nonfiction pieces about the first family are covered. Contains 15,000 words plus illustrations

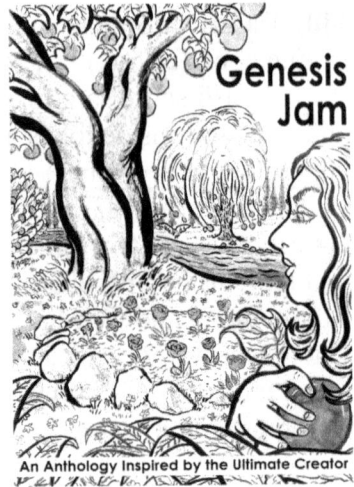

Genesis Jam

An Anthology Inspired by the Ultimate Creator

Rescuing Supermom

By Denise Chiappetta (eBook)

Essays, poetry, and comics to enrich a mother's soul. It's chick lit with true grit! Erma Bombeck meets Mary Magdalene and the result might be Denise Chiappetta. Motherhood, sisterhood, womanhood and wife-hood come under the crosshairs of an author who strives to be her best for God and family. Contains 19,000 words by Denise, and 24 comics and illustrations by Joe Chiappetta

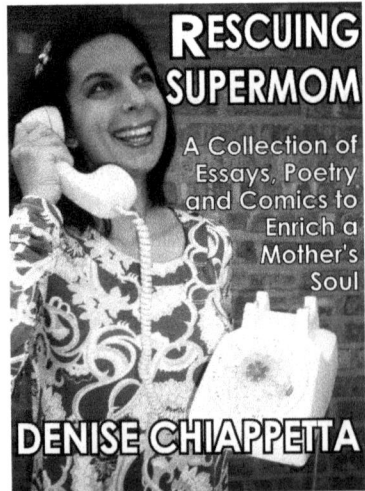

RESCUING SUPERMOM

A Collection of Essays, Poetry and Comics to Enrich a Mother's Soul

DENISE CHIAPPETTA

Silly Daddy 2004 graphic novel

Imagine Van Gogh with a wife and kid today: that's Silly Daddy. Parenting has rarely been more profound. Cartoonist Joe Chiappetta turns autobiographical storytelling into a family odyssey of road trips, break-ups, romance, sci-fi adventure, big laughs, deep thoughts, and redemption. 254 pages

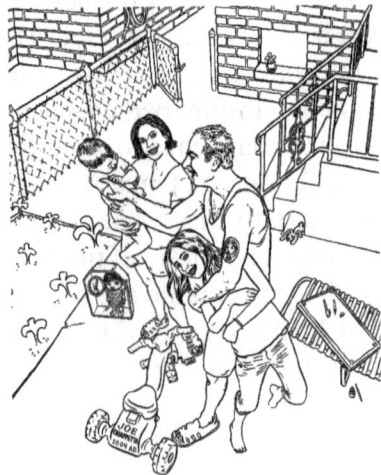

www.joechiappetta.blogspot.com

168

www.ingramcontent.com/pod-product-compliance
Lightning Source LLC
Chambersburg PA
CBHW061723020426
42331CB00006B/1064